DIV for the Superparanoid

How to perform direct intravenous ozone injections on yourself safely and confidently

by

Paola Dziwetzki

DIV for the Superparanoid
How to perform direct intravenous ozone injections on yourself safely and confidently

Copyright © 2022 by Paola Dziwetzki

Second edition, January 2022

ISBN: 9798553845551

All rights reserved. No part of this book may be reproduced in any manner whatsoever without written permission except in the case of brief quotations embodied in critical articles and reviews.

Photographs Copyright ©
Paola Dziwetzki, Michael A. Nelson, Promolife

Many thanks to Michael who was of great help in editing and proof-reading the manuscript and who gave me great tips on how to further improve it.

Thank you to Gary and Teresa for checking for errors and typos.

Content

CONTENT	1
DISCLAIMER	5
GLOSSARY	6
1. WHY I DECIDED TO WRITE THIS BOOK	7
2. WHY IS IT CALLED "DIV FOR THE SUPERPARANOID"?	8
2.1. What does DIV stand for?	8
2.2. What makes "DIV for the Superparanoid" safe?	8
Chapter 2 questions	9
Sources	9
3. RISKS OF DIV OZONE INJECTIONS	10
3.1. Death	10
3.2. Loss of consciousness	11
3.3. Paralysis	12
3.4. Phlebitis	12
3.5. Chest tightness	12
3.6. Loss of vision	13
3.7. Allergic reaction	13
Chapter 3 questions	13
Sources	13
4. CONTRAINDICATIONS: WHEN NOT TO PERFORM DIV	14
Known contraindications	14
4.1. Ventricular septal defect	14
4.2. Hyperthyroidism	14
4.3. Transplanted organs	14
4.4. Emergency situations	15
4.5. Phlebitis	15
4.6. Internal bleeding	15
4.7. Allergic reaction	15
Theoretical contraindications:	16
4.8. G6PD deficiency	16
4.9. Eosinophilia	17
Additional considerations:	17
4.10. Inability to follow instructions	17
Chapter 4 questions	17
Sources	17
5. REQUIRED EQUIPMENT	18

5.1. Oxygen tank	18
5.2. Oxygen Regulator	21
5.3. Ozone Generator	23
5.4. Syringe filling station	23
5.5. Syringe	24
5.6. Filter	25
5.7. Butterfly needle	26
5.8. Silicone tubing	26
5.9. Luer lock connectors	26
5.10. Sterile syringe caps	27
5.11. Alcohol wipes	27
5.12. Cotton pads	27
5.13. Tourniquet	28
5.14. Tape	28
5.15. Bandaid	28
5.16. Sharps bin	29
5.17. Book, smart phone, or tablet	29
Chapter 5 Questions	29
Sources	30

6. GENERAL PREPARATIONS — 31

6.1. How to set up your equipment	31
6.2. Insert a filter into the oxygen line	31
6.3. Familiarize yourself with the syringe filling station	31
6.4. Hygiene	33
6.5. Wear loosely fitting clothes	34
6.6. Make sure to be undisturbed	35
6.7. Reclined body position	35
Chapter 6 questions	36
Sources	36

7. HOW TO CREATE AN AIRTIGHT OXYGEN CIRCUIT — 37

7.1. Silicone tubing	37
7.2. Luer lock connectors	39
7.3. How to create an airtight oxygen circuit	40
Chapter 7 questions	43

8. HOW TO HANDLE AN OXYGEN TANK — 44

8.1. Fixate it	44
8.2. Keep away from heat	44
8.3. Keep away from oils	45
8.4. Half a turn to open	45
8.5. Do not exert too much pressure	46
8.6. Inspection every 5 years	46
8.7. Get a wrench	46
8.8. How to purge the regulator	46
Chapter 8 questions	47

Sources	47
9. VEINS	**48**
9.1. Which veins can be injected?	48
9.2. How to inject a vein	50
9.3. How to inject a rolling vein	51
9.4. How to prevent and treat phlebitis	52
9.5. How to make veins visible	53
Chapter 9 questions	54
Sources	54
10. "DIV FOR THE SUPERPARANOID"	**55**
Step-by-step procedure	55
Chapter 10 questions	74
Sources	75
11. HOW TO INJECT MORE THAN 60 CC	**76**
Step-by-step procedure	76
Chapter 11 questions	79
12. HOW TO TREAT VARICOSE VEINS WITH DIV INJECTIONS	**80**
Special considerations	80
Before / After Pictures	81
Chapter 12 questions	83
13. HOW TO PERFORM DIV WITH A GLASS SYRINGE	**84**
Step-by-step procedure	85
Chapter 13 questions	98
14. TROUBLESHOOTING	**101**
14.1. Chest tightness and cough	101
14.2. Trouble finding a vein	102
14.3. Blockage	102
14.4. Burning sensation	103
14.5. Crunchiness around injection site	104
14.6. Allergic reaction	104
14.7. Loss of consciousness	104
Chapter 14 questions	105
Sources	106
15. THINGS YOU SHOULD NEVER DO	**107**
15.1. Do NOT get up too early	107
15.2. Do NOT perform the injection while standing up	107
15.3. Do NOT inject too quickly	107
15.4. Do NOT skip any steps	108
15.5. Do NOT put oil around the plunger of the syringe	108

15.6. Do NOT push through the chest tightness	108
15.7. Do NOT reuse needles	108
15.8. Do NOT be lax on hygiene	108
15.9. Do NOT continue if you are unsure about steps taken	108
15.10. Do NOT push the plunger of the syringe with the tourniquet on	109
15.11. Do NOT use 55 mcg/ml for non-varicose veins	109
15.12. Do NOT use oxygen if you are not sure about its purity	109
15.13. Do NOT do DIV if you don't feel confident	109
15.14. Do NOT experiment	109
Chapter 15 questions	110

16. WHERE TO BUY THE EQUIPMENT — 111

Discount codes	111
16.1. "The Power of Ozone DIV Package"	112
16.2. Oxygen tanks and regulators	112
16.3. Ozone generators	113
16.4. Supplies	114
Chapter 16 questions	114

17. HOW TO USE DIV THERAPEUTICALLY — 115

General recommendations	115
DIV for infections	115
DIV for auto-immune conditions	116
DIV for treating varicose veins	117
DIV for treating cancer	117
DIV as a preventive measure	118
Chapter 17 questions	118
Sources	118

18. HOW TO DEAL WITH HERXHEIMER REACTIONS? — 120

Chapter 18 questions	121
Sources	121

19. HOW SAFE ARE DIV OZONE INJECTIONS? — 122

When was the first DIV ozone injection performed?	122
How many DIV injections are being performed safely?	122
How does the risk from DIV ozone injections compare with other interventions?	124
Chapter 19 questions	125
Sources	125

20. ANSWERS — 126

Disclaimer

DIV ozone injections have led to death, loss of consciousness, paralysis, and loss of vision in the past. Consequently, many professional medical ozone associations prohibit their use.

This book is not to be misunderstood as an encouragement to ignore those prohibitions and regulations. Its main purpose is to inform and educate interested readers.

I do not assume any liability or responsibility for any loss, damage, or injury caused or alleged to be caused directly or indirectly by the information, correct or incorrect, contained in or omitted from this book.

This book is sold with the understanding that the author and publisher are not liable for misunderstanding, misinterpretation, misuse or misapplication of the information provided.

The DIV method described in this book is in my opinion the safest there is, but it does not eliminate all risk. The safety of DIV ozone injection hinges on the correct application of the safety precautions and on the purity of oxygen in the oxygen tank. Both are handled by humans, and human error can never be completely eliminated.

The intention of this book is not to encourage any illegal behavior, nor to substitute professional medical advice. Use of the information in this book is at the sole risk of the reader.

The content of this book reflects my current understanding and research on the topic and may differ from my earlier or future publications.

Glossary

cc	cubic centimeter = ml = milliliter
DIV	direct intravenous ozone injection
i.v.	intravenous
IV	an intravenous injection, push, or a drip
ml	milliliter = cc
mcg/ml	micrograms per milliliter, which is the commonly used unit for ozone concentration, and is the same as mg/l, mcg/cc, or ug/cc, colloquially called "gamma"
LPM	liters per minute, unit for oxygen flow

1. Why I decided to write this book

If you have read the disclaimer, you may be shocked: death, paralysis, loss of vision due to direct intravenous ozone injections? If that's the case, why am I making such dangerous information available to a wider audience?

Yes, people have died in the past due to DIV ozone injections, but also due to drinking water, after chiropractic adjustments, taking over-the-counter medication, or simply from eating food. As a matter of fact there are more well documented cases of fatalities due to water ingestion than due to any type of ozone therapy, including DIV.

There are many misconceptions about DIV ozone injections which I hope to clarify in this book. And I hope to contribute to their safety by laying the needed precautions all out in the open, instead of having people rely on often contradictory word-of-mouth information or Youtube videos.

Thanks to my situation I am uniquely equipped for this job:

- I've been performing intravenous ozone injections for over 11 years
- I am a licensed alternative health care provider
- I used to work at a doctor's office in the "lab" where my main job was to draw patients' blood
- I completed numerous ozone therapy courses
- I am licensed in oxyvenierung, the German art of injecting pure oxygen intravenously

But probably the most fateful circumstance is the fact that I happen to own one of the few remaining copies of Dr. Hans Wolff's book "Das medizinische Ozon". It has never been translated into English. But thanks to the fact that I speak German fluently, I can read and understand it perfectly and so can make its information available to the English speaking ozone community.

Dr. Wolff's book is the key to the many myths and misconceptions about the dangers of DIV ozone injections, which I explain in chapters 3 and 19.

DIV ozone injections keep growing in acceptance and popularity. The enthusiastic promotion of DIV ozone injections by a number of ozone practitioners during the Coronavirus plandemic has led to an increased interest in this type of ozone treatment. This calls for an affordable, comprehensive, easy to understand guide for how to perform direct intravenous ozone injections in the safest possible way.

This is what I hope this book will accomplish.

2. Why is it called "DIV for the Superparanoid"?

"DIV for the Superparanoid" is a unique method I developed to perform DIV ozone injections in the safest way possible. It is the culmination of 11 years of practice and research, and it keeps improving constantly.

The name is based on the fact that the technique contains a generous overabundance of safety precautions. Some DIV experts will likely find many of the steps unnecessary and exaggerated, which is the whole point of this program.

By being "super paranoid", one uses the imagined worst case scenario to anticipate any possible risk and implements steps to actively prevent it. This method teaches confidence through proactive overcautiousness.

2.1. What does DIV stand for?
DIV is part of ozone therapy and it stands for direct intravenous injection of ozone.

During DIV, an ozone/oxygen gas mix is directly injected into the vein at a low speed of 1 cc per 10 to 30 seconds with a 27 gauge butterfly needle. The ozone/oxygen gas mix consists of 1 to 3% ozone and 97 to 99% pure oxygen.

2.2. What makes "DIV for the Superparanoid" safe?
Every step of this method is based on the following four tenets:

1. **Ozone is heavier than air.** Consequently, ozone should be handled like a liquid once the syringe is filled. Incorrect handling could lead to a spillage of the gas and a contamination with air.

2. **The injection of air into the vein has to be avoided at all costs**, since it's nitrogen which carries the greatest risk of embolism. Air consists of around 80% nitrogen. This means that all space between the oxygen tank and the needle needs to be flushed with pure oxygen before the injection.

3. **It takes a while for oxygen to be absorbed by red blood cells.** This fact dictates the speed of the injection. If the DIV is performed too quickly, there is more gas in the bloodstream than can be bound by the red blood cells and serious problems can arise, like embolisms.

4. **Gas rises in the bloodstream to the highest point, the brain.** Which means that the patient has to remain immobile and horizontal for at least 30 minutes until all the gas bubbles have dissolved. This single precaution is able to prevent most serious complications after DIV ozone injections.

Although the "DIV for the Superparanoid" method has been created to keep the risk of accidents at an absolute minimum, **it does not completely remove all risk.** So, even if all safety precautions are maintained and respected, unforeseen complications can still arise.

Chapter 2 questions

1. What are DIV ozone injections?
2. How does one gain confidence through paranoia with the "DIV for the Superparanoid" method?
3. List the four tenets upon which the "DIV for the Superparanoid" method hinges on.
4. Name the two key points why it is important to remain immobile and horizontal for at least 30 minutes after the DIV ozone injection.

Sources

[1] Scheel, Paul: "Die Transfusion des Blutes und Einsprützung der Arzneyen in die Adern. Historisch und in Rücksicht auf die practische Heilkunde bearbeitet", 1828
[2] Cole, Frank: "Intravenous Oxygen", 1950
[3] Damiani, E. et al: "Exploring alternative routes for oxygen administration", 2016
[4] Wolff, Hans: "Das medizinische Ozon", 1979
[5] "Air or gas embolism", NHS, UK
[6] Bocci, Velio: "Ozone, a New Medical Drug", 2005

3. Risks of DIV ozone injections

When it comes to DIV ozone injections, there appear to be two extreme camps in the world of ozone therapy: one group gets apoplectic seizures at the mere mention of gets apoplectic seizures at the mere mention of direct intravenous injections with ozone. The other group appears to be oblivious to risks, up to the point of negating the possibility of any gas embolism, even when air is injected.

Both groups constitute extremes and both are wrong.

Yes, there are considerable potential risks when doing DIV ozone injections, here is a list of the most drastic ones:

1. death
2. loss of consciousness
3. paralysis
4. loss of vision

All of those have taken place after DIV injections in the past. Consequently, one should employ the utmost care to prevent risks from occurring. (See chapter 14.)

Let's look at the most serious, potential problems one by one.

3.1. Death
This is the most serious and the most often evoked risk of DIV ozone injections. Among ardent promoters of DIV, death is regarded as an impossible outcome. Yet, history teaches us otherwise and proves that the injection of a pure ozone/oxygen mix can indeed lead to a deadly gas embolism.

The German cluster
In the 1970s and 1980s several deaths occurred in Germany after DIV ozone injections. The injections were performed by medical and alternative practitioners who used a unique form of direct ozone/oxygen injections. All cases have been well documented by Wolfgang Eisenmenger in the book "Outsider Methods in Medicine".

There, a total of 6 deaths are described which occurred after various ozone administrations. One of the fatalities happened after a subcutaneous injection, one was due to an intra-arterial injection, and one happened 3 weeks after a DIV injection and was officially listed as death due to pneumonia.

Three of the six are confirmed to have happened after DIV ozone injections. It's possible that an additional two of the six also passed away because of the intravenous administration of the gas. So, in total between three and five people died within a relatively short time span in a single country after DIV ozone injections.

It appears that neither before nor afterwards has a similar cluster of cases occurred anywhere else in the world, although DIV kept being practiced throughout the years. This begs the question: What did the Germans do that caused deaths after DIV ozone injections which others did not do?

As I laid out in my blog article "Can DIV ozone injections lead to death?", this was most likely due to a unique DIV method which was introduced by Dr. Hans Wolff, the leading ozone therapy expert in Germany at that time.

Dr. Wolff's unique method consisted of injecting the gas with the tourniquet firmly on the patient's limb. Something which is never performed with any medication during intravenous drug administration. The standard i.v. procedure dictates to release the tourniquet before the medication is pushed into the vein.

Dr. Wolff's technique reversed those steps. His method was devised to prevent gas embolisms, but it resulted in having exactly the opposite effect of what it intended.

Las Vegas
An often referenced case when discussing dangers of DIV ozone injections is the report of the death of an elderly woman at the hands of two men in Las Vegas.

According to the media, two men who had claimed to be doctors, met up with two women, a mother and daughter, in a private apartment. Both women received an "octozone" treatment. Both were fine and alive after the first injection.

The next day the daughter apparently administered another infusion on her mother who then lost consciousness and collapsed. An ambulance was called and she was transported to the hospital where she died a few days later.

Although it is very much possible that this is a case of death due to DIV ozone injections, the circumstances do not allow for a clear conclusion.

The procedure did not take place in a formal setting, like a doctor's office or a clinic, and the witnesses contradict each other. Since the two men denied having performed the procedure, there is uncertainty about what really happened.

3.2. Loss of consciousness
Another possible complication is loss of consciousness which can occur when the gas is injected too quickly, in too large amounts, if air is injected instead of pure

oxygen/ozone, or if the patient is not allowed to rest for a sufficiently long time afterwards.

In most cases loss of consciousness is transitory, and the person does not suffer any long term ill effects. In extreme cases it can lead to death, paralysis, neurological deficits, or visual disturbances, see above.

3.3. Paralysis

Paralysis is another serious complication which has been reported after ozone injections in Germany 40 years ago. It is assumed that this was mainly due to Dr. Wolff's erroneous technique. Partial paralysis, in some cases irreversible, has occurred in patients after both intravenous and intra-arterial injections.

Gas embolisms in the central nervous system can account for a number of serious side effects including memory loss, confusion, cognitive impairment, and speech problems.

The cause is likely the same as when loss of consciousness occurs: too much gas was injected too quickly and the patient did not remain in a reclined and relaxed position for a sufficiently long time afterwards.

3.4. Phlebitis

Vein inflammation is also called phlebitis and it is a common event after DIV ozone injections.

The injection of ozone gas, especially in too high concentrations, irritates the vein walls. They become hard, red, painful, and swollen. If this happens repeatedly, it can lead to sclerosed veins which are very difficult or impossible to puncture in the future.

3.5. Chest tightness

Chest tightness is the sensation of heaviness in the lungs, also described as the feeling of not being able to take a deep breath.

The tightness can be exceedingly painful at times. Usually, it passes within 30 to 60 minutes after the injection, although in some cases the discomfort can last for several days. This symptom can also be observed during the art of oxyvenierung, which is the intravenous administration of pure oxygen.

It's assumed that this is due to a stimulation of the endothelin peptide which causes vasoconstriction and micro embolisms in the lungs. It is important to stop the injection at the first signs of the chest sensation.

3.6. Loss of vision

This is another potential complication after intravenous ozone injections which is most likely due to gas entering the cranium and causing embolisms in sensitive capillaries.

Visual disturbances after DIV ozone injections can happen in patients with a history of ocular migraines. They are often temporary and the patient regains the sight within hours. In more severe cases (see the German cluster) loss of vision can be permanent.

Just as with other serious complications, a slow and safe administration with at least a 30 min resting period should in most cases prevent this problem.

3.7. Allergic reaction

Full body itch, welts, redness, and swelling - these are signs of an allergic reaction which can also arise as a consequence of DIV ozone injections. In such a case it's important to not continue with the treatments to prevent a potential anaphylactic shock.

The above list is not a complete collection of potential complications and other problems which have not been mentioned here, can arise as well.

In order to see the risks of DIV ozone injections in context and to find out how often they occur, go to chapter 19.

Chapter 3 questions

1. Has it ever occurred that people died from DIV ozone injections? Please, list all the reported cases.
2. Describe Dr. Hans Wollf's flawed DIV technique and explain what made it so dangerous.
3. What is the chest tightness due to?
4. List some of the neurological symptoms which could be an indication of a gas embolism in the brain.

Sources

[1] Eisenmenger, Wolfgang: "Außenseitermethoden in der Medizin, Zur Ozontherapie", 1986
[2] Bundesgerichtshof, Urteil vom 29.01.1991, Heilpraktiker; Sorgfaltspflichtverletzung, AZ: VI ZR 206/90
[3] Dziwetzki, Paola: "Can DIV Ozone Injections Lead to Death?"
[4] Wolff, Hans: "Das medizinische Ozon", 1979
[5] thejournal.ie: "Two charged with murder after death of woman injected with oxygen in 'naturopathic' treatment", May, 2015
[6] Las Vegas Review Journal: "Two men indicted in death of 74-year-old woman", June 24, 2015
[7] Raw story: "Quack 'doctors' face murder charges after injecting air bubbles into woman's blood to 'kill pathogens'", May 7, 2015
[8] Kreutzer, Franz J.: "Intravenöse Sauerstofftherapie (IOT)", 2014

4. Contraindications: When NOT to perform DIV

There are certain conditions which are contraindicated for ozone therapy generally or for DIV ozone injections specifically. If a person suffers from one of those conditions, they should not receive DIV ozone injections or any other type of ozone therapy.

Some of them are **known contraindications** agreed upon by most ozone associations. Others are being discussed as possible, or what I call **theoretical contraindications**, since there is no evidence that they in fact lead to complications after ozone treatments, but it can't be excluded that they could do so in the future. I include both in this list.

Known contraindications
Most ozone experts agree to not administer DIV ozone in the following cases:

4.1. Ventricular septal defect
A ventricular septal defect is a hole in the heart between the left and right heart chamber. In a healthy human being the two chambers are separated by a wall. This prevents the venous and arterial blood from mixing.

In an individual with a septal defect the oxygen/ozone bubbles during a DIV injection could enter the arterial bloodstream and then find their way into the brain. This could result in neurological deficits (see chapter 3) and even death.

Patients with VSD should not receive DIV ozone injections.

4.2. Hyperthyroidism
Ozone is believed to stimulate hormone production. In patients who suffer from hyperthyroidism, ozone treatments could trigger a thyrotoxic crisis.

There are a number of diseases which can cause the body to produce too much thyroid hormone, like Graves' disease, Plummer's disease, or thyroiditis. If they are not well controlled through medication, an ozone treatment should not be performed.

4.3. Transplanted organs
It has been observed that ozone therapy can be a great immune system stimulator. This can be a problem for people who have a transplanted organ like a heart, kidney, liver, or a lung from a donor.

People with transplanted organs are required to take immunosuppressive medication to prevent their bodies from rejecting the foreign organ. Ozone treatments, working exactly opposite of immune system suppressive drugs, could trigger an organ rejection.

4.4. Emergency situations

Any type of emergency situation like a heart attack, stroke, internal or external bleeding, physical trauma (accident), or an asthma attack are also contraindications for DIV ozone injections. In all those cases 911 should be called immediately.

4.5. Phlebitis

Phlebitis is the inflammation of the vein, something which often occurs during DIV ozone injections. If your vein is red, painful, hard, and swollen after the last DIV treatment, give it time to rest and heal before you puncture it again. Do not perform DIV on an inflamed and swollen vein.

4.6. Internal bleeding

Ozone treatments are known to render red blood cells more flexible, which can lead to an improved blood circulation. Something which is undesirable if there is bleeding present.

Menstrual bleeding is not regarded as a contraindication.

4.7. Allergic reaction

Patients can develop allergic reactions to DIV ozone injections. Something which I didn't believe for the longest time, but it seems that my Dad is such a case, see pictures below.

It appears that this is not a reaction to ozone, but a reaction specifically to DIV ozone injections, since he is responding well to ozone saunas and breathing ozone bubbled through olive oil.

Symptoms of an allergic reaction to a DIV injection can be: a full-body itch, redness, welts (even on limbs which have not been injected), and swelling.

It can be difficult to distinguish an allergic reaction from phlebitis or a Herxheimer reaction. If you are unsure about what is going on, do not continue with the DIV treatments.

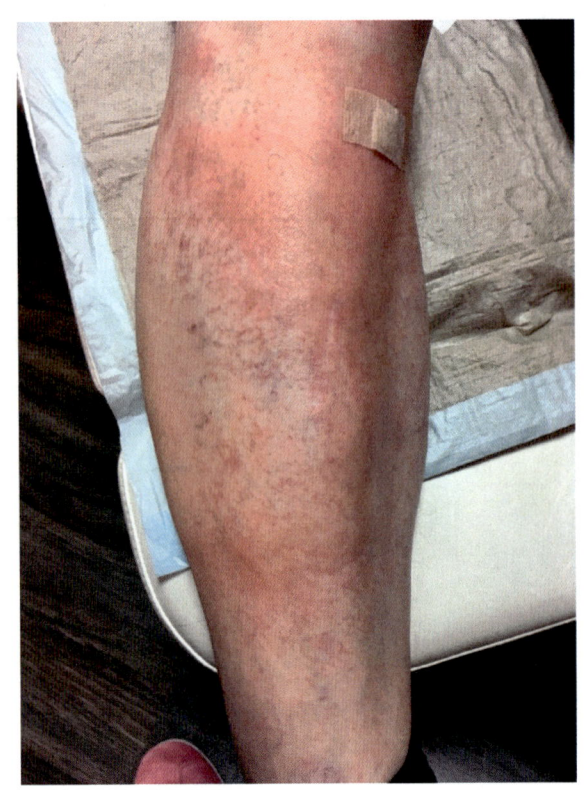

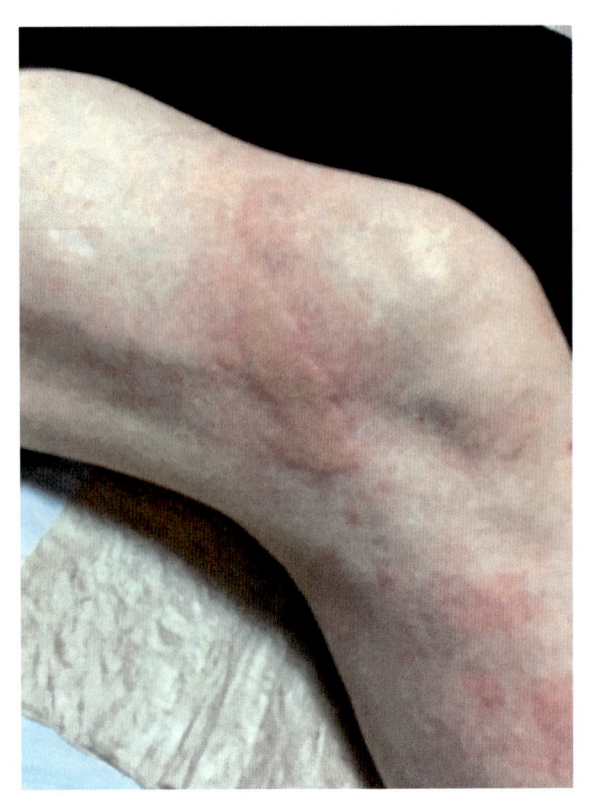

Pictures of my Dad after a DIV ozone injection. See the welt like swelling on the right, and the swelling and redness on the left. I believe that these are symptoms of an allergic reaction.

Theoretical contraindications:

These are considerations where ozone therapy could pose a problem, although there are no documented cases where this ever happened.

4.8. G6PD deficiency

G6PD is an enzyme which is important for the production of glutathione, a potent antioxidant. If there is not enough G6PD, not enough glutathione can be produced to counteract the reactive oxygen species which are introduced during ozone therapy, so goes the argument. Theoretically, this could lead to uncontrolled bleeding, as is sometimes observed during vitamin C administration in G6PD deficient patients.

But: there is no known case of anyone having had an adverse reaction after ozone therapy because of G6PD deficiency.

G6PD deficiency occurs at higher rates in people with Mediterranean, Asian, Middle Eastern, or African origin. Given that ozone therapy is highly popular in India and many Asian countries and in Italy and Spain, it is possible that this is not a real concern. But it may make sense to keep it in mind and to proceed cautiously in cases with a known G6PD deficiency.

4.9. Eosinophilia

The injection of pure oxygen intravenously is known to lead to elevated eosinophils, a certain type of white blood cells. This has been well documented after oxyvenierung, the injection of pure oxygen intravenously.

If the patient already suffers from chronically elevated eosinophils (eosinophilia), a further increase could have negative consequences. Although eosinophilia is not mentioned as a contraindication for oxyvenierung.

Additional considerations:

4.10. Inability to follow instructions

Some people have difficulties following instructions. Reading and understanding guidelines and being able to follow them are critical skills to be able to learn how to do DIV ozone injections. If you have problems adhering to directions, you should not attempt intravenous ozone injections.

Chapter 4 questions

1. List all the known and theoretical contraindications for ozone therapy.
2. Why should ozone treatments not be performed on people with transplanted organs?
3. How could a ventricular septal defect cause a complication with DIV ozone injections?

Sources

[1] Mayo Clinic: "Hyperthyroidism (overactive thyroid)"
[2] Renate Viebahn-Hänsler: "Ozon-Sauerstoff-Therapie", 2009
[3] Bocci, Velio: "Ozonization of blood for the therapy of viral diseases and immunodeficiencies. A hypothesis"
[4] healthline.com: "About Immunosuppressant Drugs"
[5] Kreutzer, Franz J.: "Intravenöse Sauerstofftherapie (IOT)", 2014
[6] Dziwetzki, Paola: "Do You Need a Test for G6PD Deficiency Before Ozone Therapy?"
[7] G. Douglas Campbell jr.: "Ascorbic Acid-Induced Hemolysis in G-6-PD Deficiency", 1975
[8] Quinn, Joseph: "Effect of High-Dose Vitamin C Infusion in a Glucose-6-Phosphate Dehydrogenase-Deficient Patient", 2017
[9] Mayo clinic: "Ventricular septal defect (VSD)"

5. Required equipment

The "DIV for the Superparanoid" method calls for certain types of equipment and supplies which other DIV methods do not require. The right type of equipment is critical for the safe administration of ozone injections.

To find out where you can buy all the supplies discussed in this chapter, go to chapter 16.

5.1. Oxygen tank

The safety of DIV ozone injections largely hinges on the quality of oxygen which should be of at least 99% purity.

Only oxygen from certain types of oxygen tanks satisfies this requirement. Those are:

- Medical tanks (CGA 870 and CGA 540)
- Ultra high purity, scientific grade oxygen tanks (CGA 540)
- Promolife's O2Ready tanks

Every tank requires a matching low flow, or a so-called pediatric regulator. A CGA 870 tank calls for a matching CGA 870 low flow regulator. A CGA 540 tank calls for a matching CGA 540 low flow regulator, just as an O2Ready tank requires a special low flow regulator.

A tank without a low flow regulator cannot be used for ozone therapy purposes.

Oxygen tanks come in different sizes. A tank which holds a few hundred liters of gas will last a year or longer if it's used only for DIV injections.

Oxygen concentrators and other types of oxygen tanks should not be used for the "DIV for the Superparanoid" method or any other type of DIV.

A tank holds oxygen under extreme pressure, which requires certain safety precautions to avoid accidents.

5.1.1 Medical oxygen tank

In order to obtain medical oxygen, most gas suppliers will ask for a prescription from your doctor. Although there are now exceptions in certain states.

Medical oxygen tanks hold oxygen of around 99.5 to 99.9% concentration. Smaller medical tanks are equipped with a CGA 870 valve which can come either as a straight post or with a toggle.

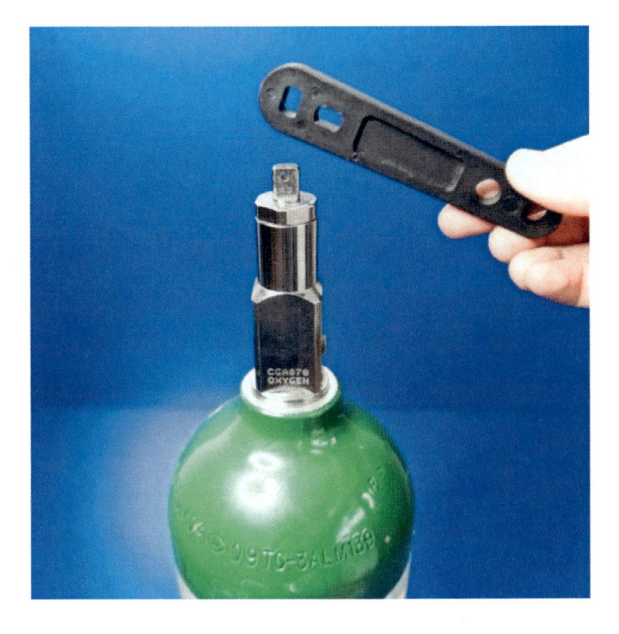

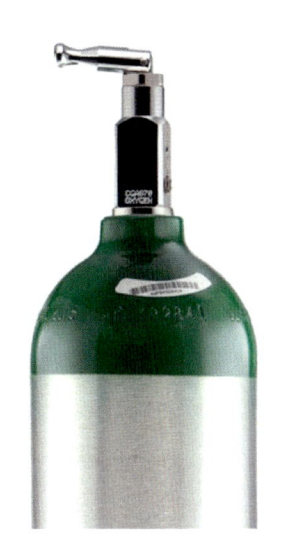

This is a medical tank with a CGA 870 straight post valve. It requires a wrench to open.

This is a medical tank with a CGA 870 toggle valve. It does not require an additional wrench to open.

A size D medical tank holds 425 L, a size E holds 680 L of oxygen. Given that a syringe for DIV holds 0.06 L of oxygen, a single tank can last many years. Bigger medical tanks which hold 1,700 liters of oxygen or more, come with a CGA 540 valve.

5.1.2 Ultra high purity, scientific grade oxygen tank

Ultra high purity oxygen is 99.994% pure O2, and consequently of even higher quality than medical oxygen. It's also called scientific grade oxygen.

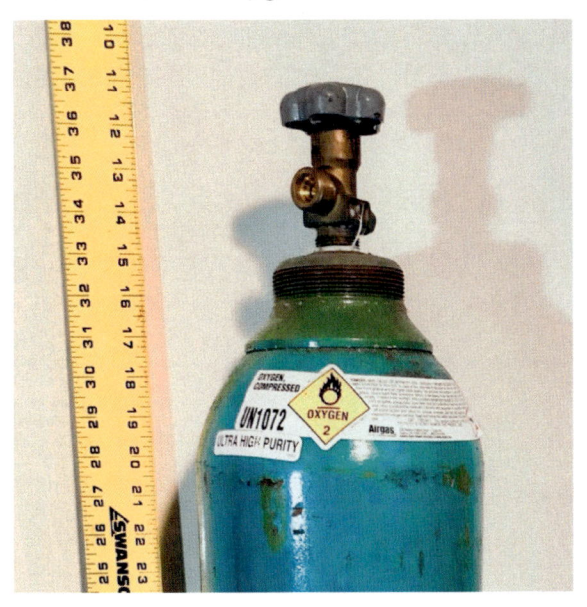

Each batch comes with a certificate of purity which proves that it has been tested.

Ultra high purity oxygen is available in big steel tanks which hold 80 CF (over 2,000 liters) of oxygen. No special license is required to obtain it.

Left, a picture of an 80 CF scientific grade oxygen tank.

Ultra high purity scientific grade oxygen tanks are equipped with an industrial CGA 540 valve which calls for a matching low flow CGA 540 regulator.

In my opinion scientific grade oxygen is currently the best type of oxygen. It's purer than medical grade, comes with a certificate that it has been tested, and does not require a prescription or a license.

5.1.3. Promolife's O2Ready pre-filled tanks

Promolife offers a unique option to obtain tanks filled with certified, high purity oxygen. If you live anywhere in the contiguous USA you can buy 99.6% pure oxygen without a prescription which will be delivered straight to your home.

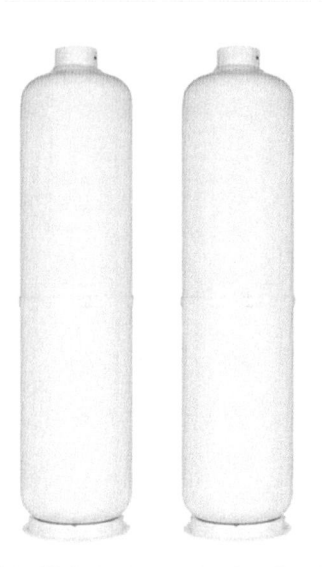

They are sold in pairs and can not be refilled. Once the tanks are empty you need to dispose of them and buy a new batch.

The tanks require a separate, unique regulator which needs to be added to the first order.

Two tanks hold together around 200 L of high purity oxygen.

A pair of Promolife's O2Ready pre-filled oxygen tanks.

5.1.4. Industrial oxygen - not recommended

Industrial oxygen is only available in CGA 540 oxygen bottles. For the longest time it was believed that industrial oxygen was of the same purity as medical oxygen, but tests by members of our ozone community have shown that this is not necessarily so.

A tank which was tested with two different analyzers turned out oxygen contents of around 96% purity. It is not clear if this was an exception or if this is a more common problem since rarely anyone tests their oxygen tanks.

An oxygen content of 96% is not pure enough to perform DIV ozone injections. At this point I do not recommend using industrial oxygen for DIV ozone injections.

5.1.5. What type of oxygen should NEVER be used

There are two types of oxygen which should never be used for DIV ozone injections: oxygen concentrators and Bernzomatic oxygen. Oxygen concentrators produce oxygen of 90 to 97% purity, but it can be also as low as 40%. None of this is sufficient for DIV ozone treatments.

An oxygen concentrator should never be used for intravenous ozone injections.

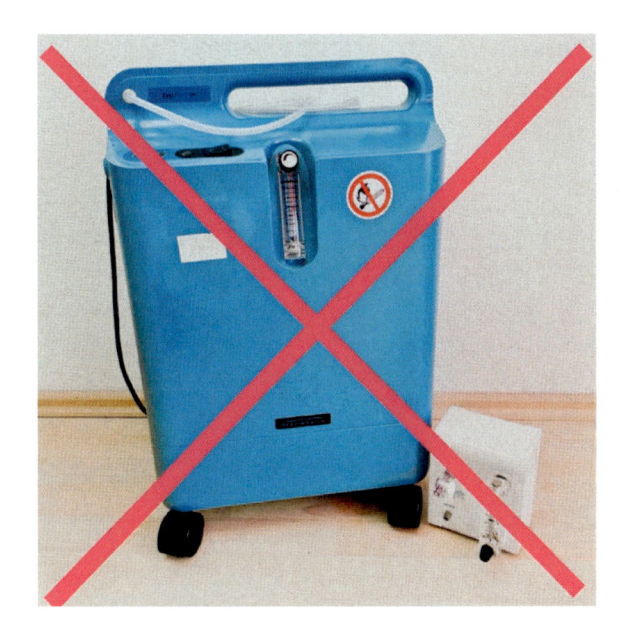

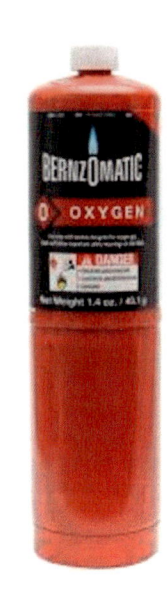

The Bernzomatic oxygen tanks hold 95% pure oxygen and are not adequate for DIV injections either.

Bernzomatic is a brand of oxygen which can be acquired at Home Depot and other home appliance shops. It consists of around 95% pure oxygen and is equally inadequate for any type of ozone injections.

5.2. Oxygen Regulator

An oxygen regulator is screwed onto the valve of the tank and controls the flow of oxygen. An oxygen tank can only be used with a matching regulator. Without it, an oxygen tank is useless.

Special low flow (pediatric) regulators are required for most ozone generators. A regulator is called low flow if it can produce flows of 1/32, 1/16, ⅛, ¼ LPM (Liters Per Minute), or similar. The flows can be also written in decimal numbers instead of fractions:

1/32	= 0.03 LPM
1/16	= 0.06 LPM
⅛	= 0.125 LPM
¼	= 0.25 LPM
½	= 0.5 LPM

The different types of oxygen tanks call for different types of regulators:
The scientific grade, ultra purity tanks require industrial CGA 540 pediatric regulators.

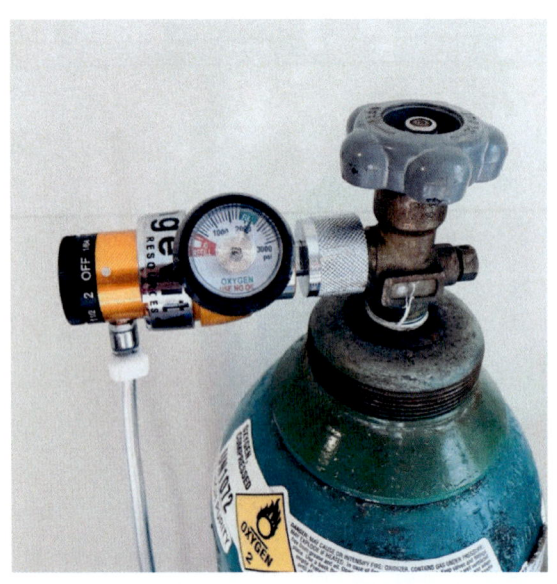

This is an ultra high purity, scientific grade oxy-gen steel tank with a CGA 540 valve and a CGA 540 low flow regulator.

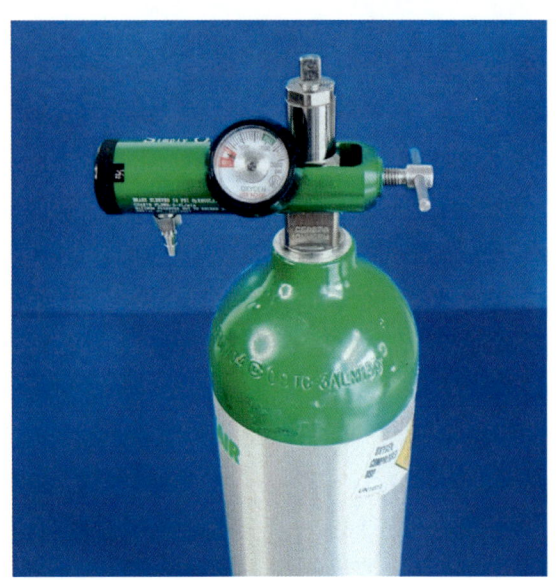

This is a medical aluminum tank with a CGA 870 straight post valve and a low flow CGA 870 regulator with a barb (not a DISS) outlet.

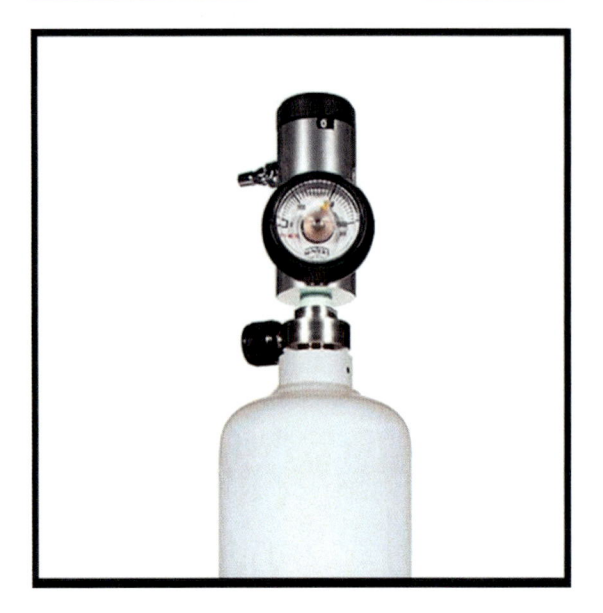

A pre-filled Promolife O2Ready tank with a matching, unique, low flow regulator.

The Stratus 3.0 ozone generator uses its own specific low flow regulators for both CGA 870 and CGA 540 tanks which have additional low flow settings.

5.3. Ozone Generator

A wide range of ozone generators can be used for DIV ozone injections. An adequate ozone machine should be able to produce ozone concentrations between 20 to 30 mcg/ml at oxygen flows of ⅛ to ½ LPM. The ozone generator cannot be an air-fed machine.

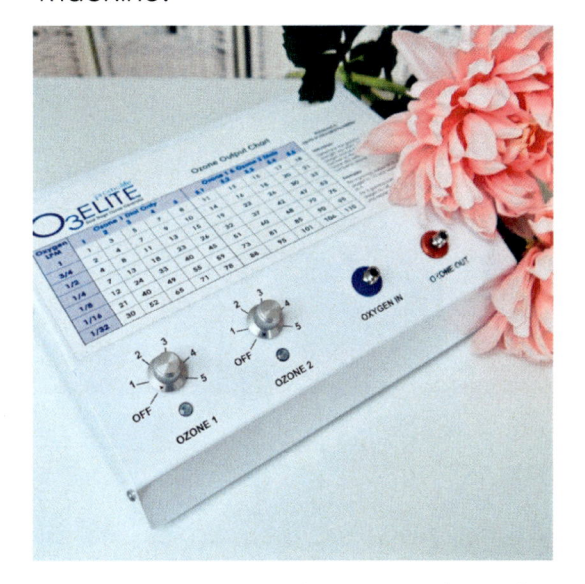

The ozone generator should also be equipped with an ozone output chart where the units of the ozone concentrations are denoted in either mcg/ml, ug/ml, mg/L, or gamma.

Any ozone generator from Promolife, Longevity, or SimplyO3 satisfies these requirements.

The Promolife Dual Cell ozone generator, my personal favorite.

Note: When ordering machines from Longevity, ask to have the standard quick attachments exchanged for luer lock connectors.

5.4. Syringe filling station

The syringe filling station is an essential part of the "DIV for the Superparanoid" program. It allows for the filling of the syringe in a way that prevents air from getting inside.

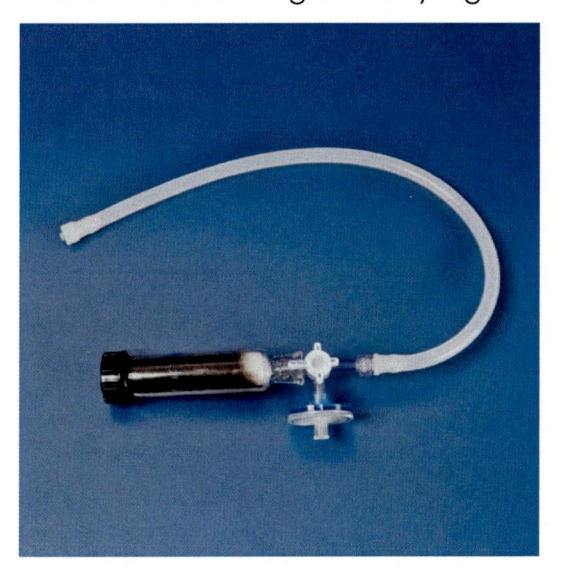

It consists of a destructor, a 3-way-valve, a filter, a piece of silicone tubing (ca. 16 inches, or 40 cm), and a luer lock connector.

Chapter 6.3. explains how the filling station works.

Left, a Promolife syringe filling station. It is part of the TPO DIV package, see chapter 16.

5.5. Syringe

There are different types of syringes which have been used for DIV ozone injections by ozone doctors or amateurs. But only one can be used for the "DIV for the Superparanoid" method: the ozone syringe.

All syringes have their pros and cons, there is no perfect solution, but the ozone syringe is still the best option, in my opinion. Here is why:

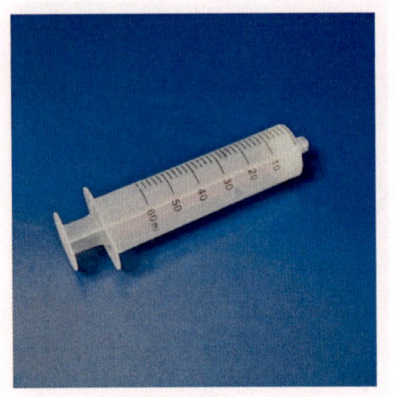

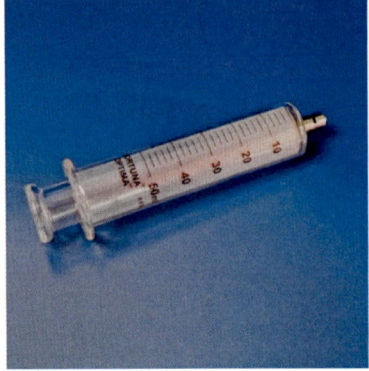

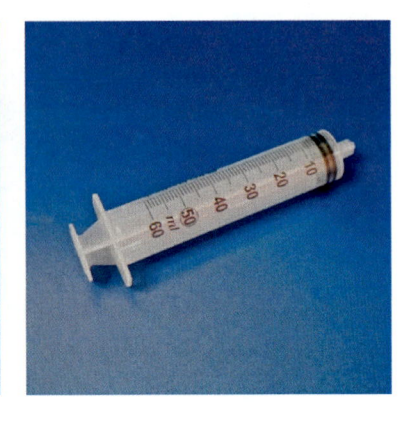

Ozone Syringe ✔

Pros:
- is made of excellent grade A ozone resistant materials: polycarbonate and silicone
- the plunger stays in place when moved
- will not break, if dropped

Cons:
- Plunger offers a significant resistance, which means it slows down the flow of oxygen and likely distorts the ozone concentration.
- markings are in 2 cc increments

➜ **CAN BE USED FOR "DIV FOR THE SUPERPARANOID"**

Glass syringe

Pros:
- completely ozone resistant material (glass)
- plunger less likely to stick or resist motion

Cons:
- Plunger can fall out of the syringe, and is more complicated to handle. The risk of mishandling the syringe and allowing air to enter is high.
- glass can break, if dropped
- markings are in 2 cc increments

Regular syringe

Pros:
- plunger stays in place when moved
- plunger less likely to stick or resist motion
- will not break, if dropped
- markings are in 1 cc increments

Cons:
- Material is not ozone resistant, neither black rubber nor plastic or syringe. Black rubber begins to leave black smears after a few uses.

The ozone syringe is made of fully ozone resistant material and has a plunger which stays in place when it is pushed.

IMPORTANT: the markings on the ozone syringe show 2 cc increments, not 1 cc. In order to inject 1 cc of gas the plunger has to be moved halfway between two different lines on the syringe.

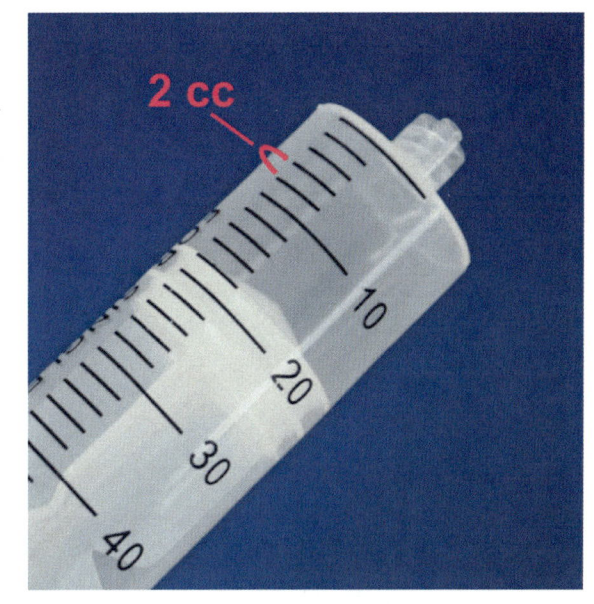

5.6. Filter

For DIV ozone injections, one filter is used at the syringe port to eliminate any contaminants and dust particles. Another one is used in the oxygen line between the O2 tank and ozone generator.

The syringe filling station already comes with a filter, so you just need an additional one for the oxygen line.

The filter is made of either PVDF or PTFE, both excellent, grade A ozone resistant materials.

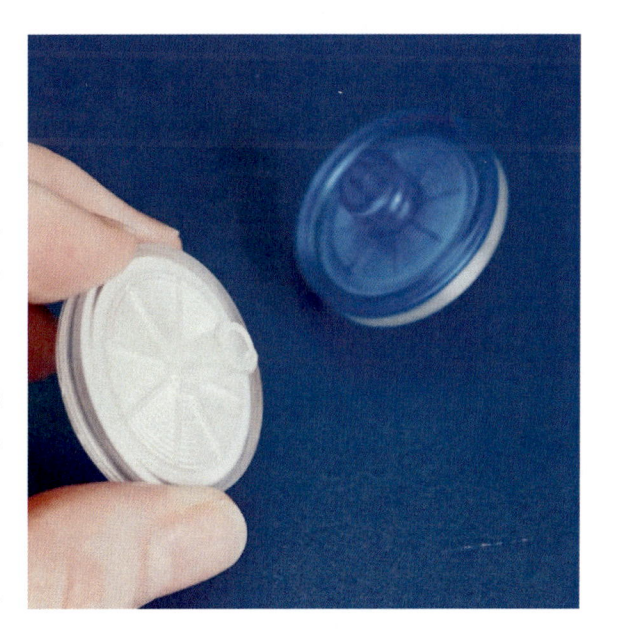

Ideally, the filter should come in single use, sterile packaging. An ozone practitioner should use a new, sterile filter for each patient. Do not confuse a filter with a check valve.

5.7. Butterfly needle

The correct needle for DIV ozone injections is a 27 gauge butterfly needle. If more than 60 cc of ozone/oxygen are injected, a 25 g butterfly needle can be used, but never bigger. The needle itself is either ½ or ¾ " long.

The diameter of the needle dictates the size of the oxygen bubbles in the vein. The bigger the gauge (g) number, the smaller the diameter of the needle and the smaller the bubbles it creates.

5.8. Silicone tubing

Around 5 feet (1.5 m) of silicone tubing are needed to connect the oxygen tank with the ozone generator.

Recommended size:
OD 5/16" x ID 3/16"
(= 0.8 x 0.5 cm)
OD = outer diameter
ID = inner diameter

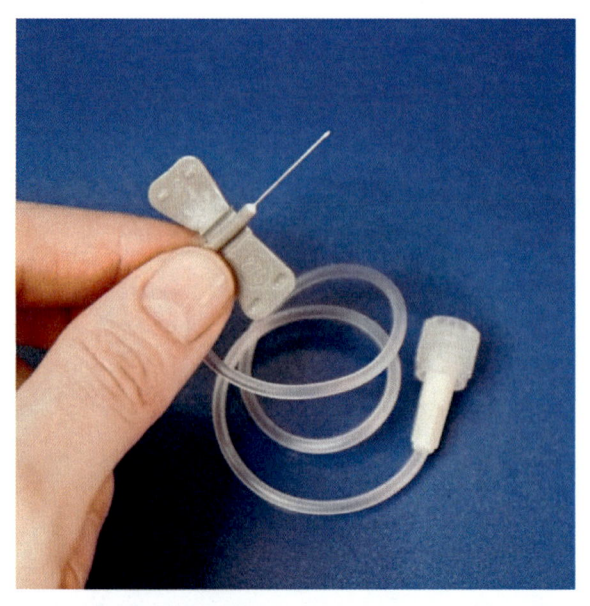

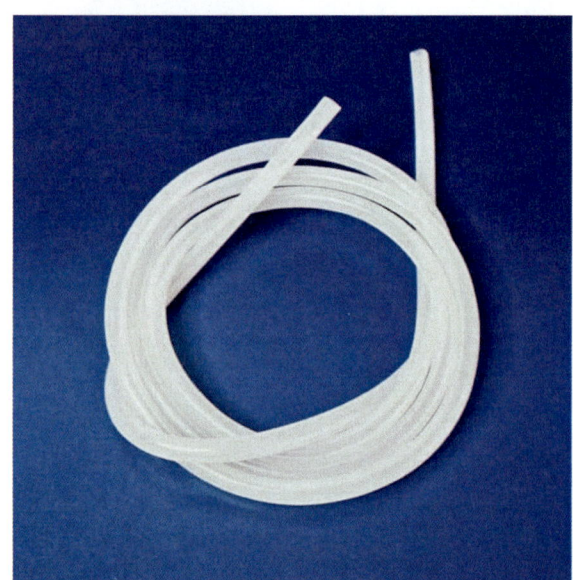

5.9. Luer lock connectors

A pair of luer lock connectors are necessary to insert the filter into the oxygen line and to connect the silicone tubing with the ozone generator.

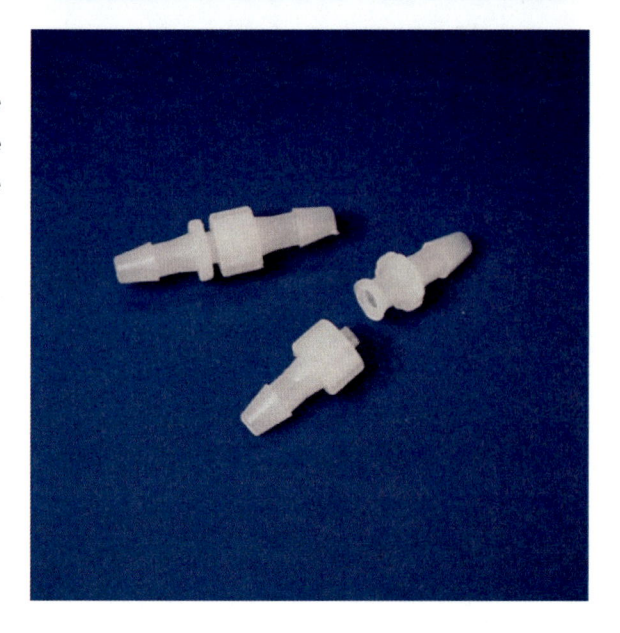

5.10. Sterile syringe caps

They keep the filling station and the syringe free of dust and dirt and are an important part of keeping everything as sterile as possible.

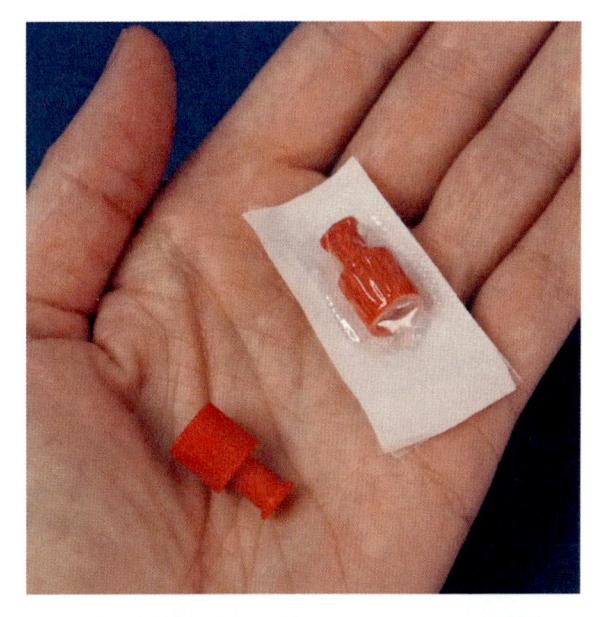

5.11. Alcohol wipes

A disinfectant is used to clean the puncture site, the filter on the syringe filling station, and the syringe itself.

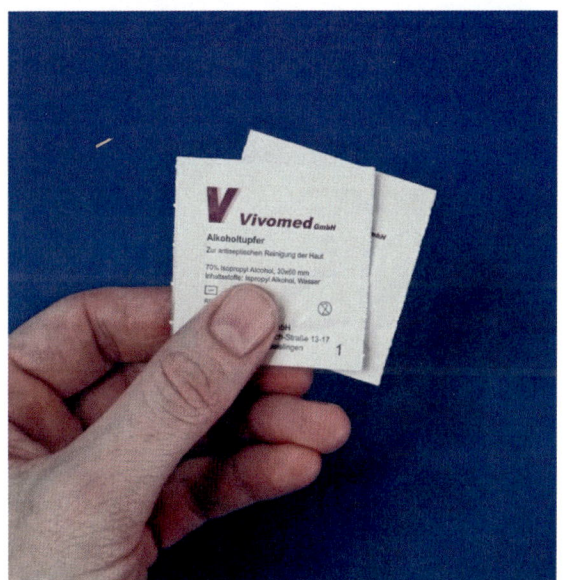

5.12. Cotton pads

Cotton, or better cellulose, pads are used to press on the puncture wound to stop bleeding after the needle has been pulled out.

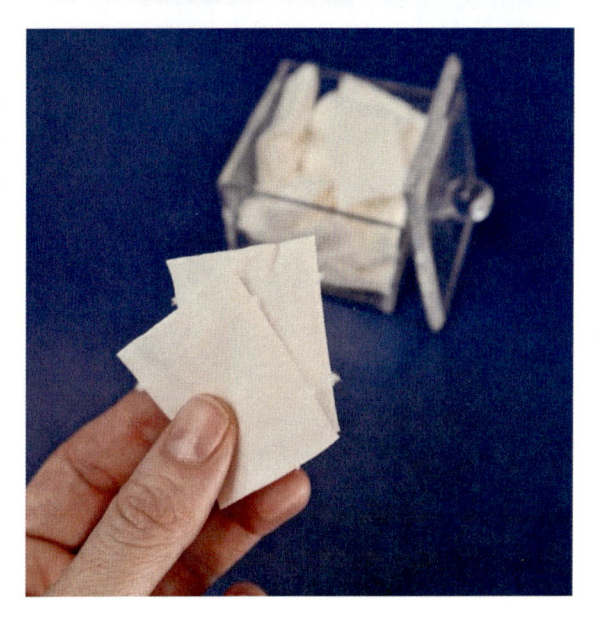

5.13. Tourniquet

A tourniquet is used to make the veins plump up and facilitate the puncturing. It should have a closing mechanism which is easy to use. Do not use single use tourniquets for self-injection.

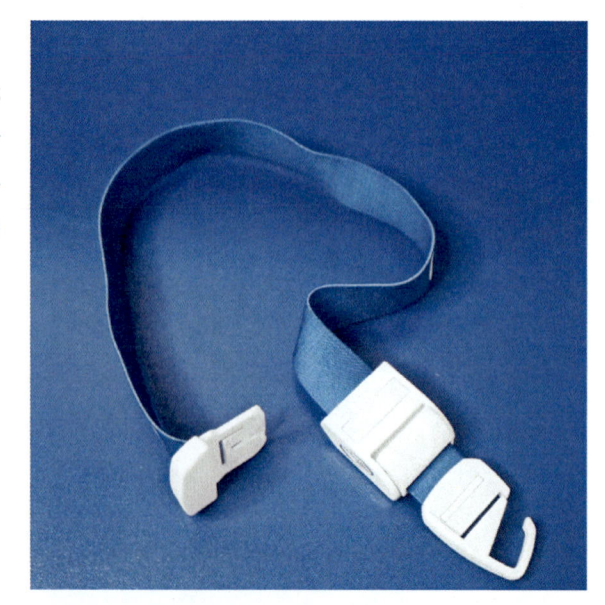

5.14. Tape

Tape is used to fixate the butterfly needle in the vein. The tape should be either transparent or 0.5" (1 cm) wide to be able to see the blood backflow in the butterfly line. When you inject someone else, the size and color of the tape does not matter.

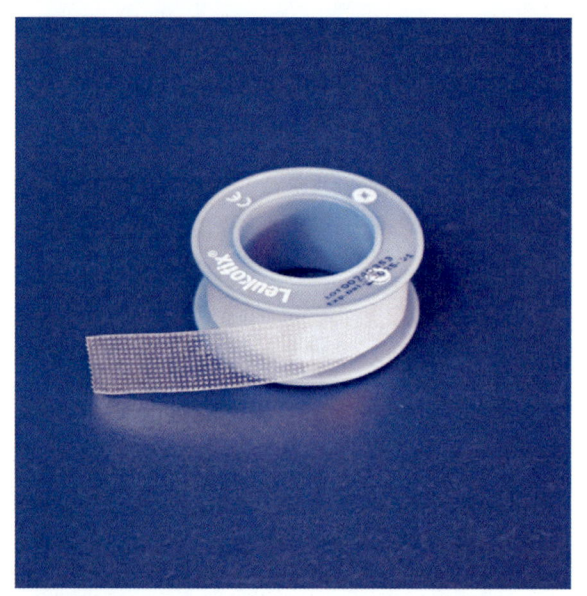

5.15. Bandaid

A band-aid is applied onto the puncture wound to stop bleeding.

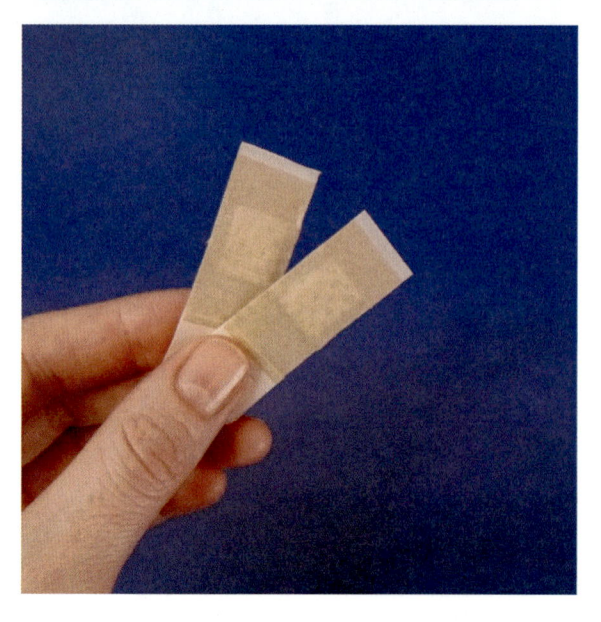

5.16. Sharps bin

A special container is used to dispose of the needles in a safe manner. Once it is full, close the lid and throw the bucket into the trash, preventing others from puncturing themselves. Alter-natively, an empty laundry bottle may be used.

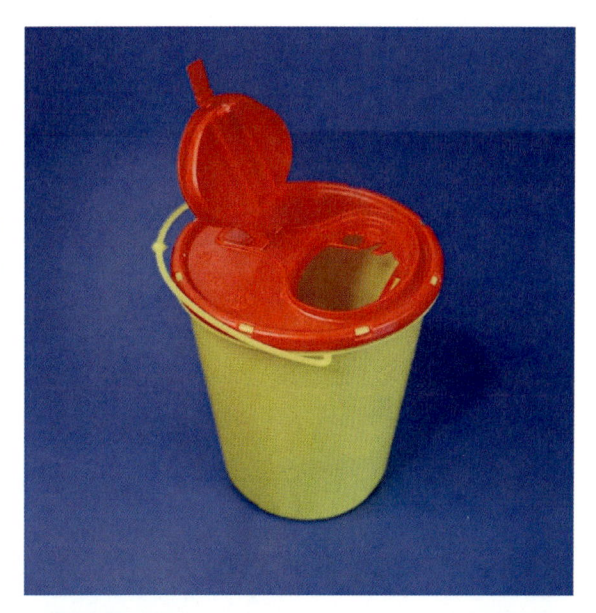

5.17. Book, smart phone, or tablet

Make sure to have something to keep yourself occupied with after the injection. You will need to remain immobile and horizontal for a good 30 minutes afterwards. Use a book, smart phone, or a tablet. Keep an eye on the clock as well.

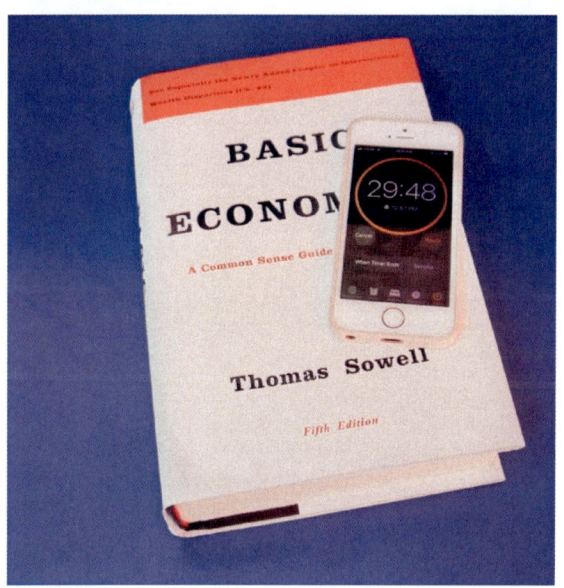

Chapter 5 Questions

1. How pure does oxygen have to be so that it can be used for DIV ozone injections (in %)?
2. Can the "DIV for the Superparanoid" technique be also performed without a syringe filling station?
3. What are the acceptable butterfly sizes for DIV ozone injections? And why?
4. Which supplies are used to keep everything as clean as possible?
5. Why is it necessary to use a special container to dispose of used needles?
6. Why does the tape have to be either transparent or 0.5 inches wide when DIV is performed?
7. What are the syringe caps used for?

Sources

[1] Applied Home Healthcare Equipment: "Oxygen cylinder sizes and info"
[2] Conversation in the Facebook group "The Ozone Group" about industrial oxygen levels (you must be a member of the group to be able to read it)

6. General preparations

There are a few general but nonetheless important considerations to undertake before starting the ozone injection. They all contribute to the safety of the protocol

6.1. How to set up your equipment

Everything should be arranged in a way that you can grab supplies with the extension of your arm without having to get up to reach for the tape or the cotton pads right after you infused the gas into your vein.

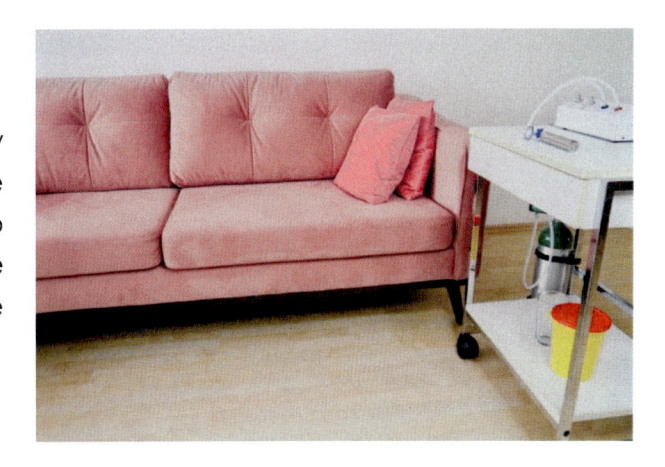

6.2. Insert a filter into the oxygen line

Insert a filter into the silicone tubing that goes from the oxygen tank to the ozone generator. The filter removes any impurities, dust, and contaminants, see chapter 7.3.

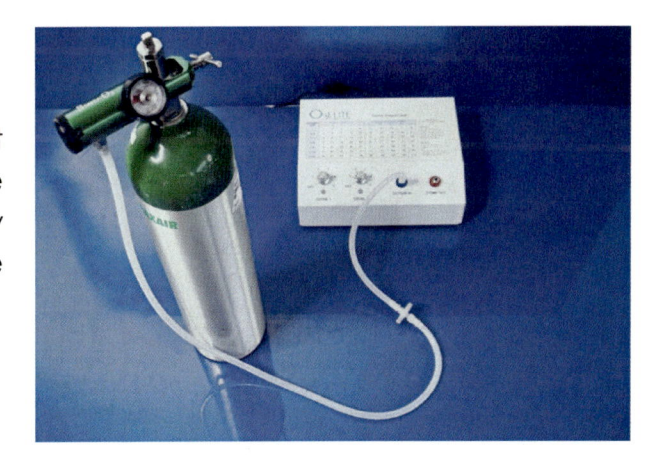

6.3. Familiarize yourself with the syringe filling station

The filling station is an important part of the "DIV for the Superparanoid" method, so it is important to understand how it works before you start the injection

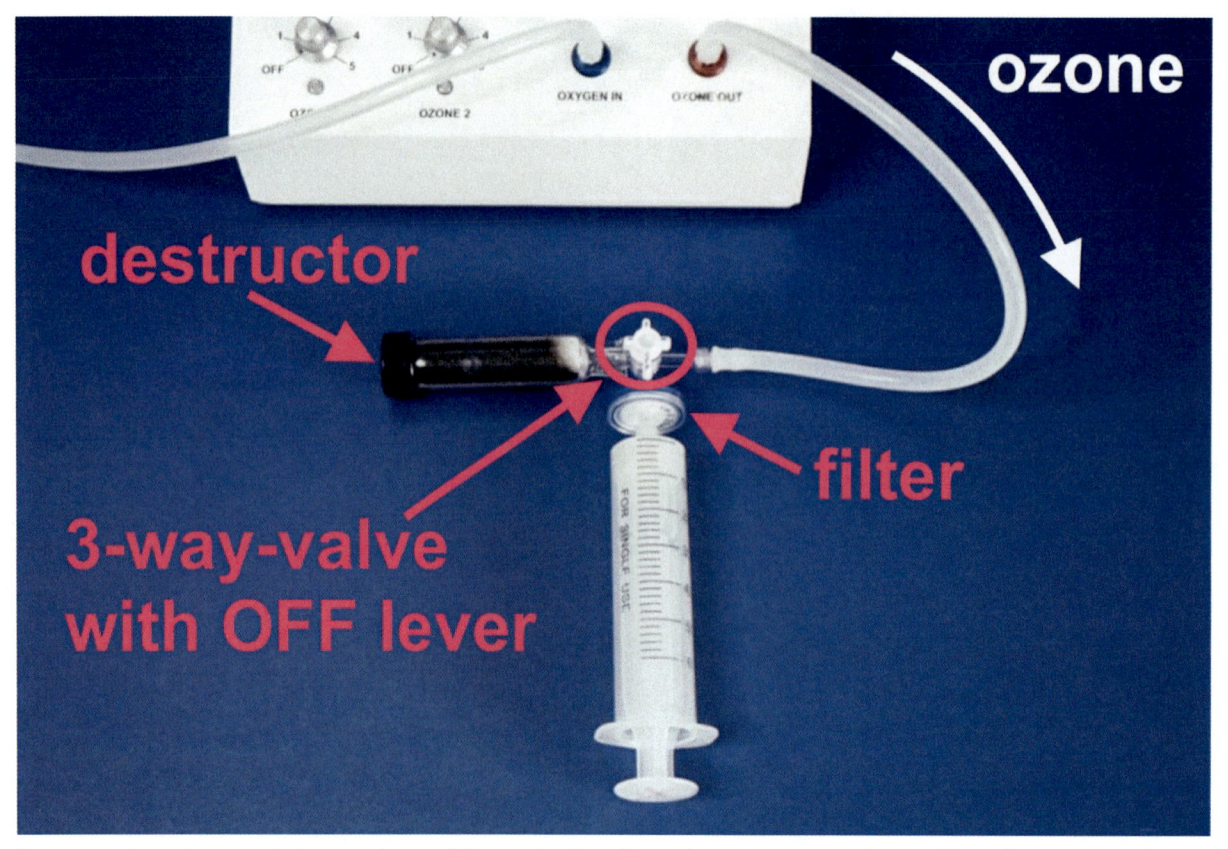

The centerpiece of the syringe filling station is a three-way-valve with a flow selector in the form of a lever marked with the word OFF. Attached to the valve are a destructor, a filter, and silicone tubing which goes to the "ozone out" port of the ozone generator.

The OFF lever can be turned either towards the destructor, the syringe port, or the silicone tubing. Whatever port the OFF lever is turned towards, it closes the gas flow towards that port.

Examples:

With the OFF lever turned towards the destructor, the ozone (white arrow) can now flow into the syringe.

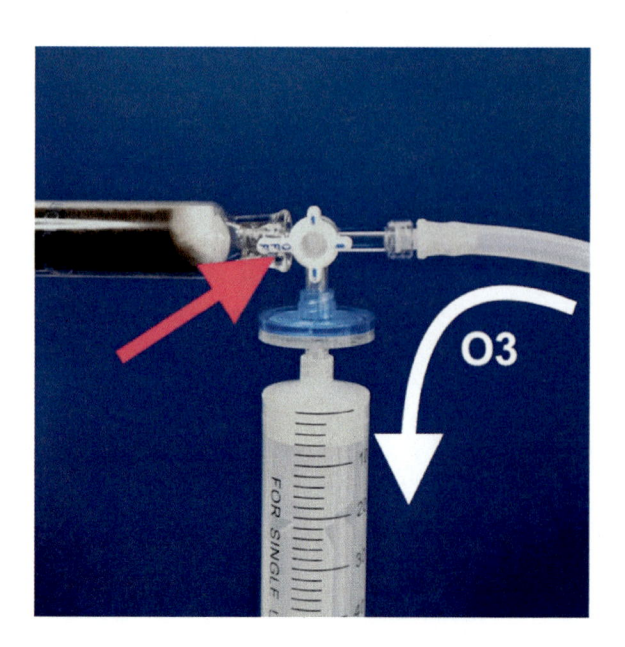

With the OFF lever pointing down towards the syringe port, the ozone will flow into the destructor.

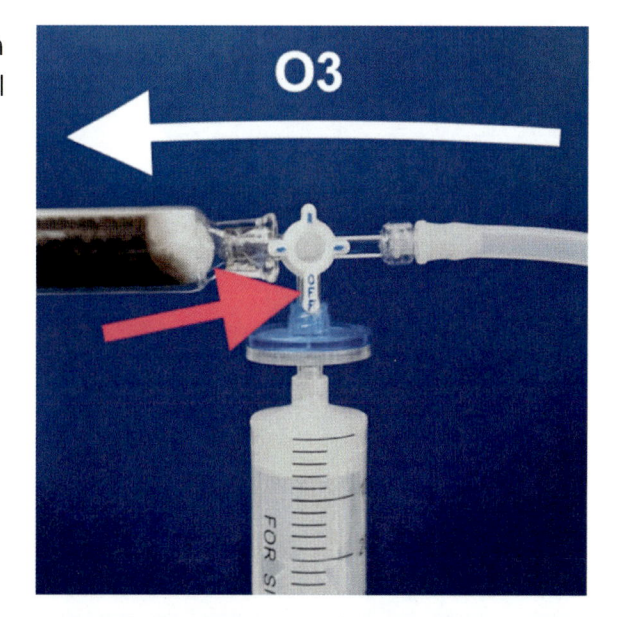

Is the OFF lever turned towards the silicone tubing, then the gas flow is blocked. Don't ever do it. Otherwise it will result in a loud popping sound and a sudden disconnect of one of the tubing.

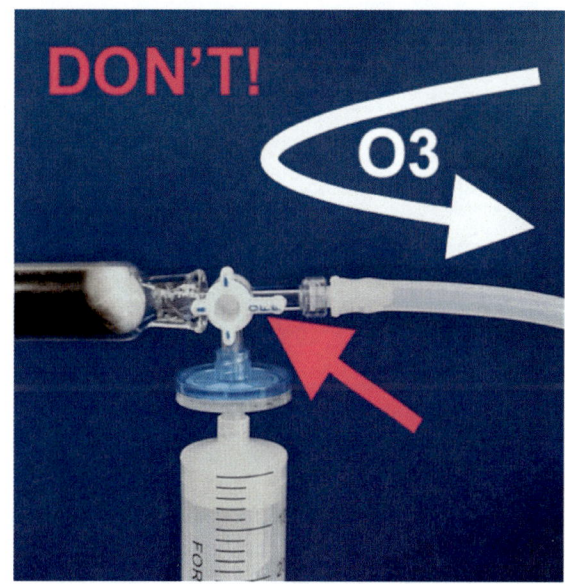

6.4. Hygiene
Always be mindful that you are introducing something into your bloodstream so you want to maintain the utmost cleanliness.

Wash your hands, make sure they are free of dirt or oil. Use a disinfectant to remove any possible pathogens. Use gloves, if you feel comfortable with them. If you do, pick them one size smaller than your hands to make them fit tightly. This will come in handy when handling sticky tape.

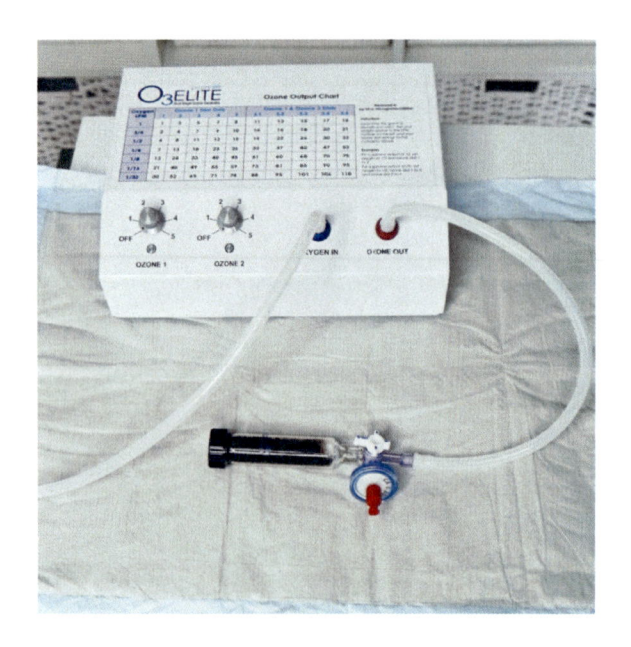

Clean and disinfect the surface of the working station. Make sure everything is free of dust and dirt.

Use a clean underpad to lay out all the supplies on.

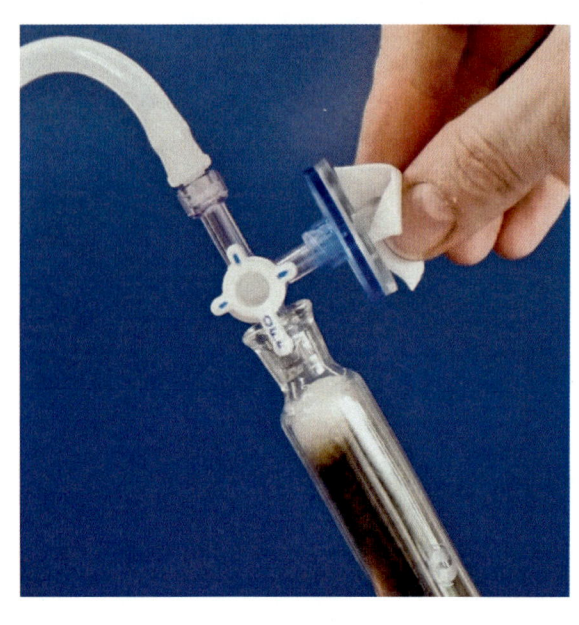

Wipe the filter with alcohol before attaching the syringe, especially when reusing the filter. Or use a new, sterile filter for each injection.

Do the same with the syringe tip, if you reuse the syringe.

Put a sterile cap on the syringe and on the filter after the injection to protect them from dust and dirt.

Use only new, sterile butterfly needles for each injection. Don't reuse them.

For medical professionals: use only **single use, disposable supplies**. This includes the syringe, the filter, and the needle, of course.

6.5. Wear loosely fitting clothes

Wear clothes which do not hinder the free circulation of blood. If you inject someone else: instruct them accordingly.

It's important that there is no obstacle for the blood to flow freely inside your body and so no possibility for a gas buildup. Such a gas buildup could, when released with a sudden move, create the same situation which has been described in section 3.1. and could lead to severe complications.

6.6. Make sure to be undisturbed

During the injection you want to be undisturbed. Calculate around one hour for the whole procedure. In that time, tell your kids to not bother you, lock your pets away, and inform your roommates or family members to give you privacy.

Don't plan the injection when you're expecting a visitor or an important phone call. Avoid situations which will require you to get up suddenly to open the door or to have a lively conversation with someone during the 30 minutes right after the DIV.

6.7. Reclined body position

Get into a stretched out and horizontal position, as far as possible. This allows the gas to linger in the bloodstream for a longer time instead of rising to the highest point, the brain (in case of an undiagnosed VSD).

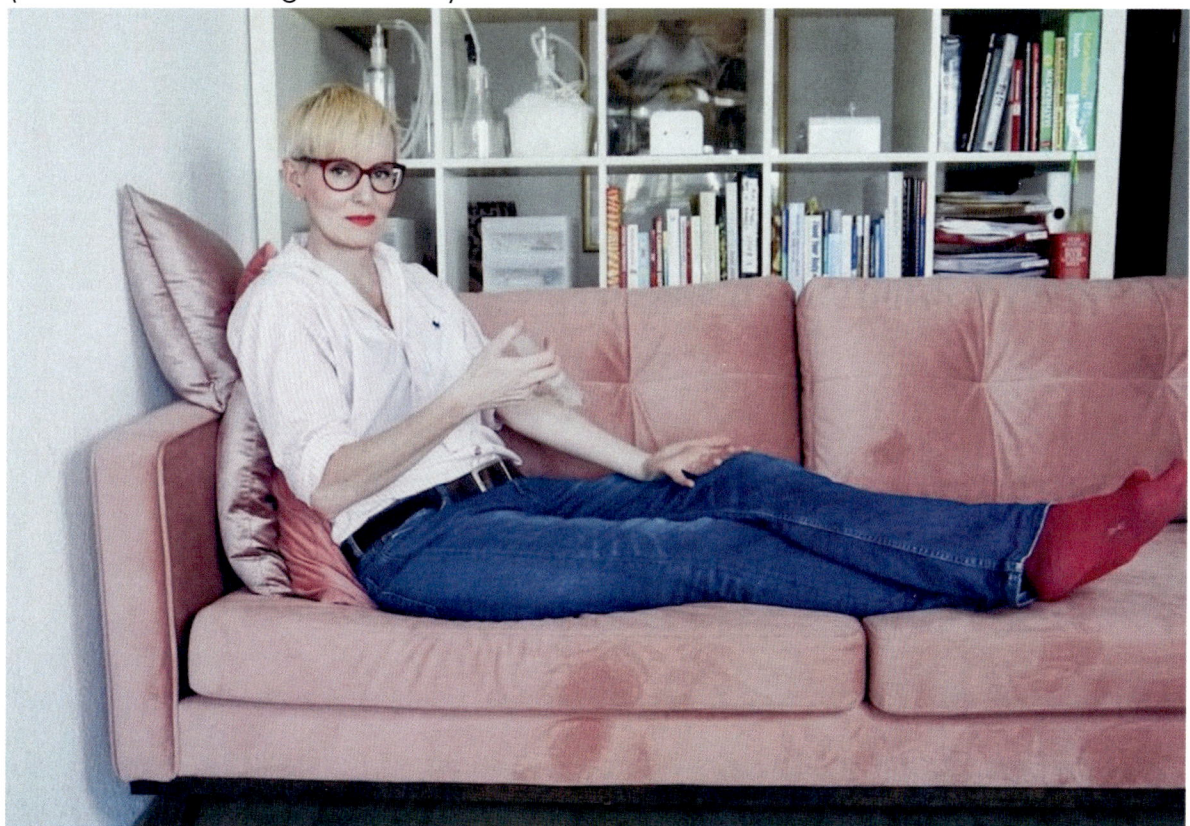

If you can recline further than shown in the picture without negatively impacting your ability to perform the injection, then do so.

Chapter 6 questions

1. Why do you want to keep supplies like tape, cotton pad, and band-aid close to where you will perform the injection?
2. Describe what to do to make sure everything is as clean and sterile as possible.
3. Why are the clothes you wear during DIV important?
4. How much time should you carve out for a DIV injection and why?

Sources

[1] Kreutzer, Franz J.: "Intravenöse Sauerstofftherapie (IOT)", 2014

7. How to create an airtight oxygen circuit

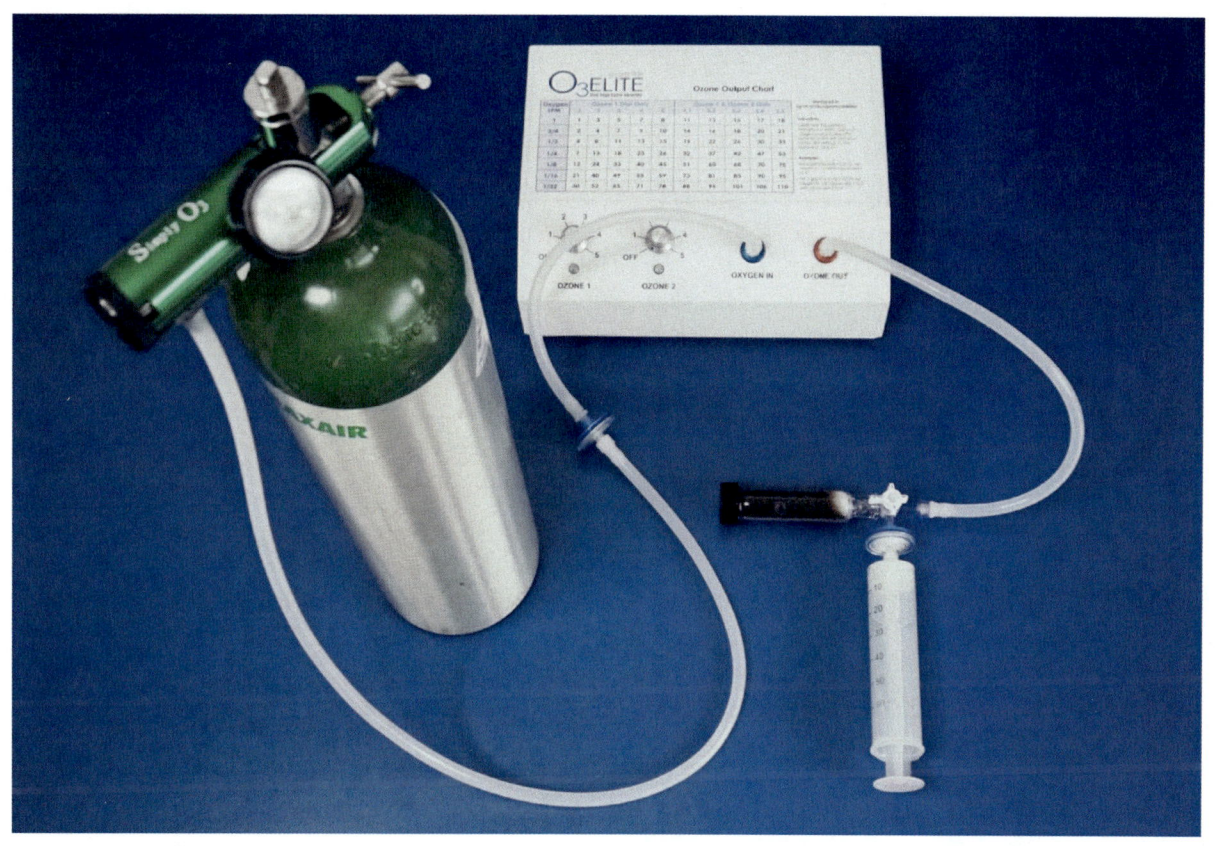

An example of an ozone setup with an airtight oxygen circuit, starting with the oxygen tank down to the syringe.

In order to perform DIV as safely as possible you have to make sure that all connections from your oxygen tank through your ozone generator all the way to your three-way-valve with your filter, destructor, and syringe connection are connected in an airtight manner without any leaks.

There are two ways to achieve this:

1. silicone tubing with the correct measurements (OD 5/16" x ID 3/16", or 8 x 5 mm)
2. luer locks

7.1. Silicone tubing
Most sellers of ozone equipment ship their ozone generators with two different types of tubing: PVC (clear) and silicone (milky colored). The PVC is typically used to transport oxygen from the oxygen source to the ozone generator, the silicone tubing is used to transport ozone gas from the ozone generator to the accessories.

37

For the "DIY for the Superparanoid" method silicone tubing is used for every connection including the path between your oxygen tank and your ozone generator. The reason for this is that silicone forms a much tighter attachment than PVC, see the pictures below.

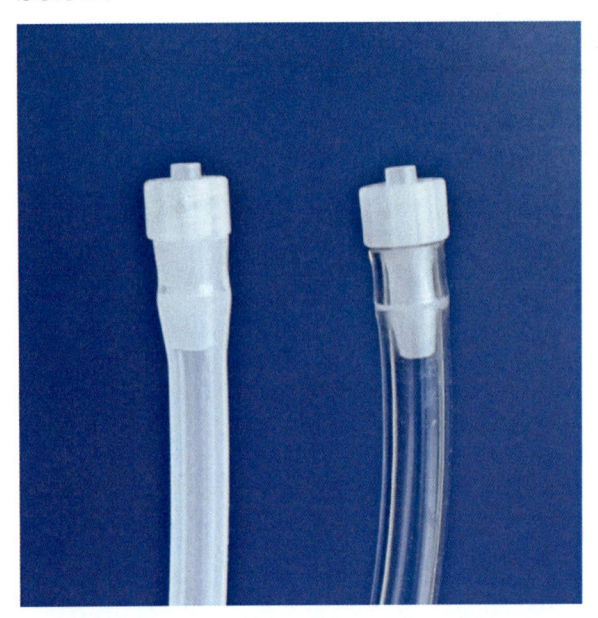

See how the silicone tubing (left) bulges over the luer lock connector indicating a tight adherence of the tubing to the connector. This is much less the case with the PVC tubing (right).

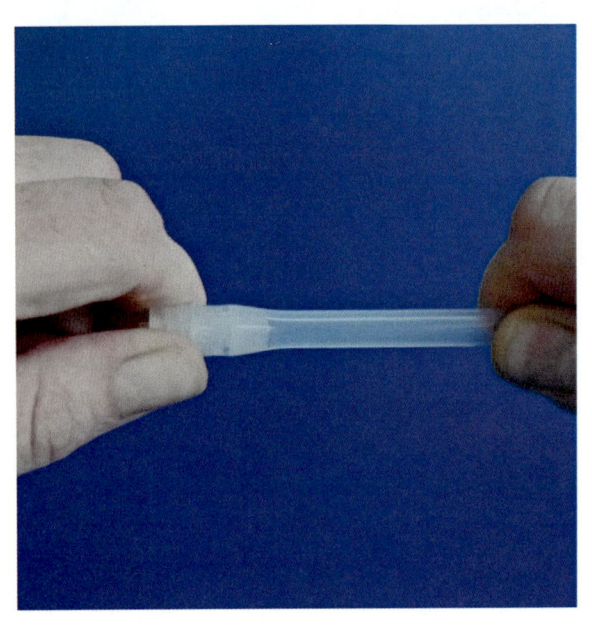

When pulling on the silicone tubing, considerable force is necessary to get it unstuck from the luer lock connector. This is a good test to verify the strength of the connection.

The following are the correct sizes for silicone tubing:
OD 5/16" x ID 3/16" (OD 8 x ID 5 mm).

Silicone hoses can become loose after a while so it's important to check them regularly. If the tubing has become loose, exchange it for fresh pieces.

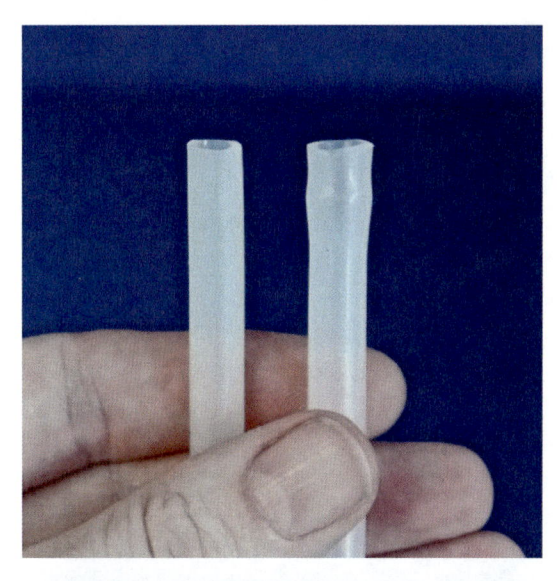

The left silicone tubing has been unused, the right contained a luer lock connector for several months. After a while this creates a deformity which can cause gas leaks.

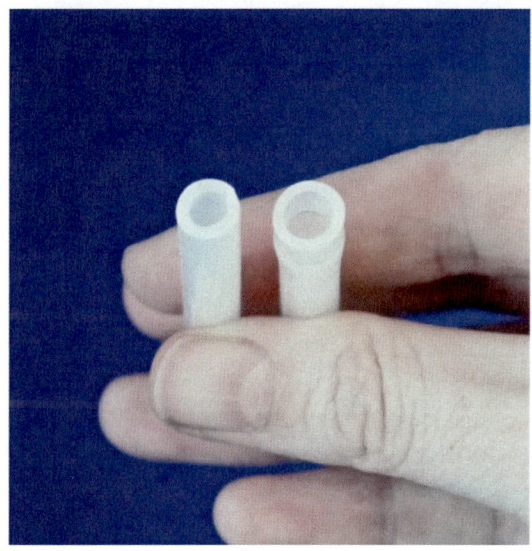

Top view: the diameter of the tubing which used to house the luer lock is wider.

Check the connections between silicone tubing and connectors regularly by pulling on them to see if they are still tight. If they come out easily, it's time to exchange the silicone for fresh pieces.

7.2. Luer lock connectors

Luer locks are universally sized mini screws which create an airtight connection. Each pair of luer locks consists of a male and a female part. Use them for all paths: to connect tubing with the ozone generator and for the syringe filling station.

Two pairs of luer lock connectors. Each pair consists of a male and a female part.

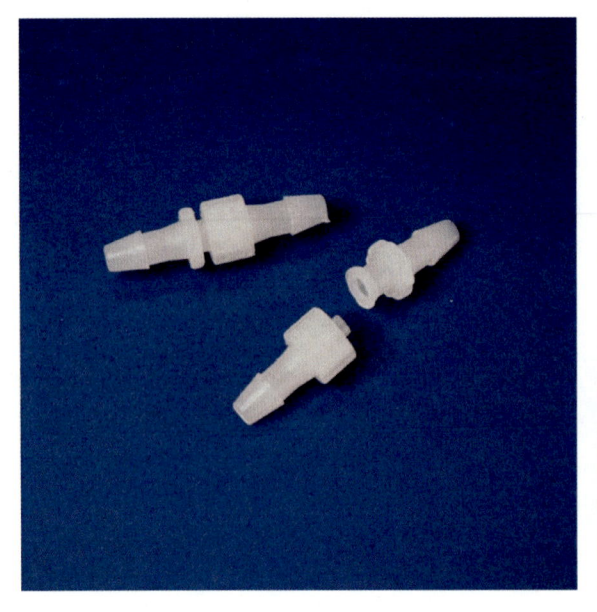

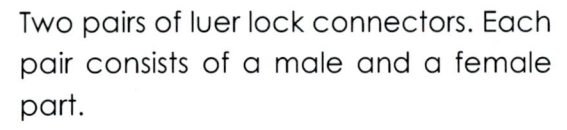

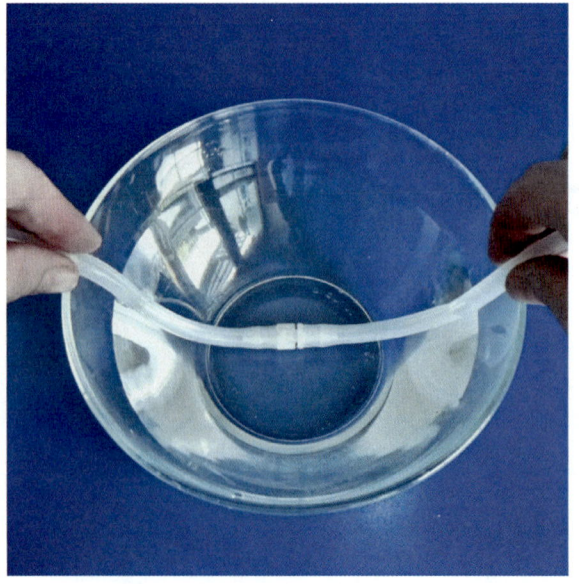

Two pieces of silicone tubing connected by a luer lock pair are submerged in water while oxygen at 5 LPM flows through them. No gas bubbles are visible - proof that the connection is completely air tight.

7.3. How to create an airtight oxygen circuit

Here are step-by-step instructions how to create an airtight oxygen circuit from the oxygen tank to the syringe filling station. A CGA 870 medical tank and regulator are used in this example.

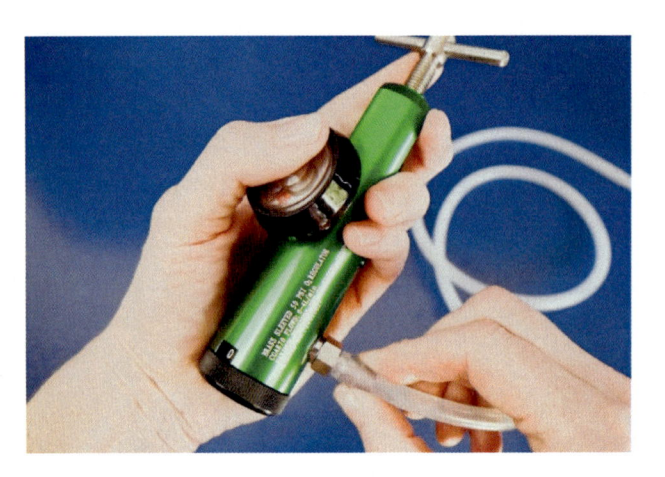

Step 7.3.1.
Take 5 feet of silicone tubing and attach it to the barb outlet of the regulator.

40

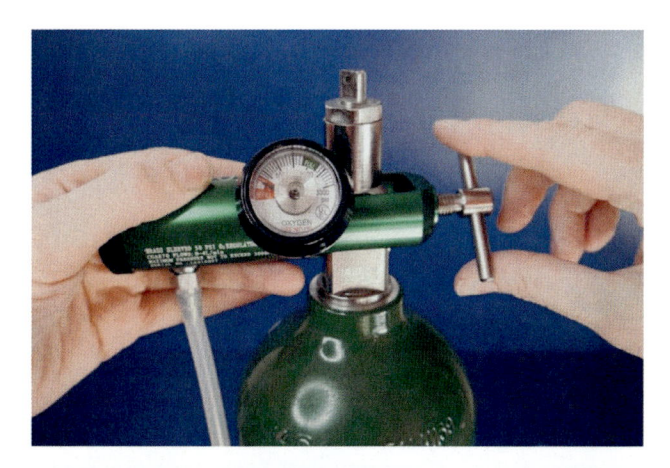

Step 7.3.2.
Screw the regulator onto the oxygen tank. Make sure it's tight.

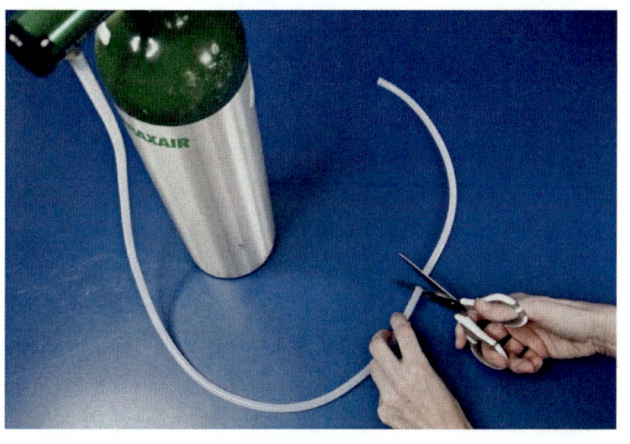

Step 7.3.3.
Cut a piece of the silicone tubing off.

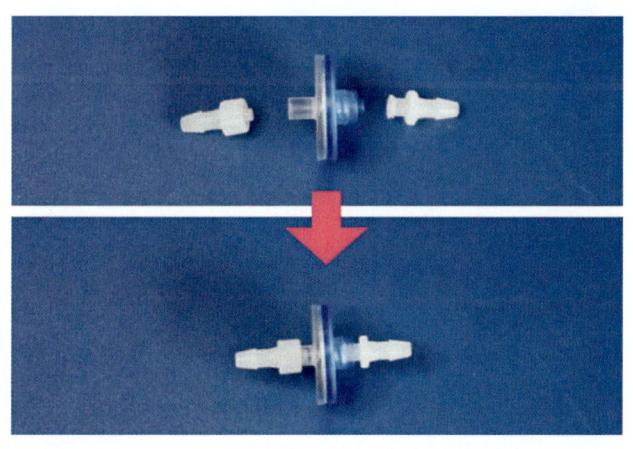

Step 7.3.4.
Attach a male and a female luer lock connector to each side of the filter.

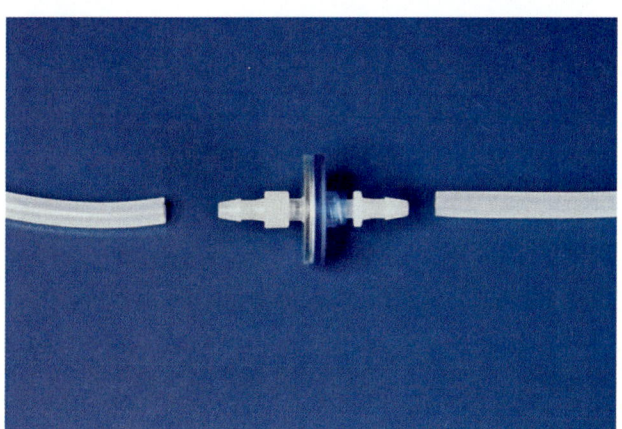

Step 7.3.5.
Connect the filter to the silicone tubing ...

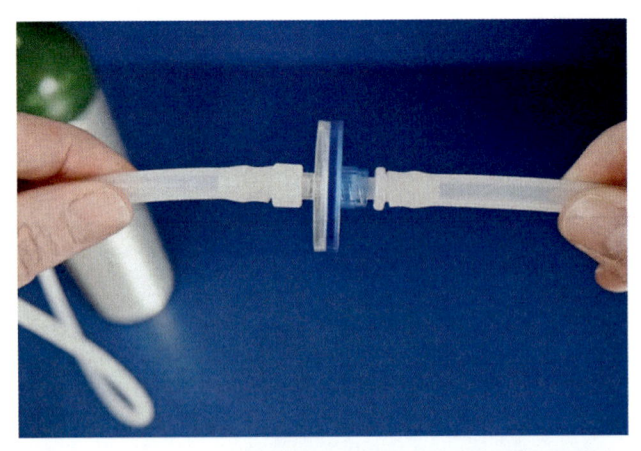

... by pushing the tubing onto the luer locks.

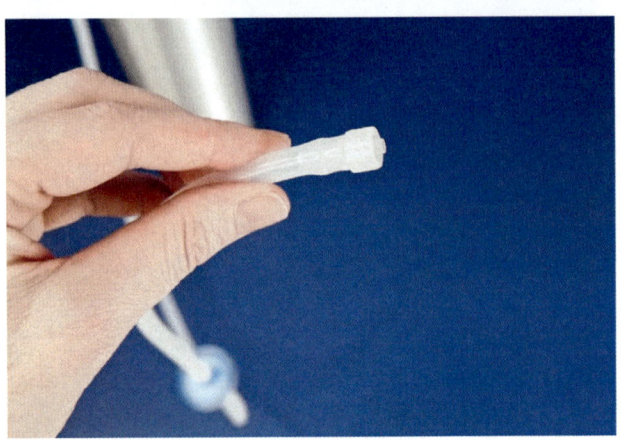

Step 7.3.6.
Take another male luer lock connector and push it into the other end of the silicone tubing.

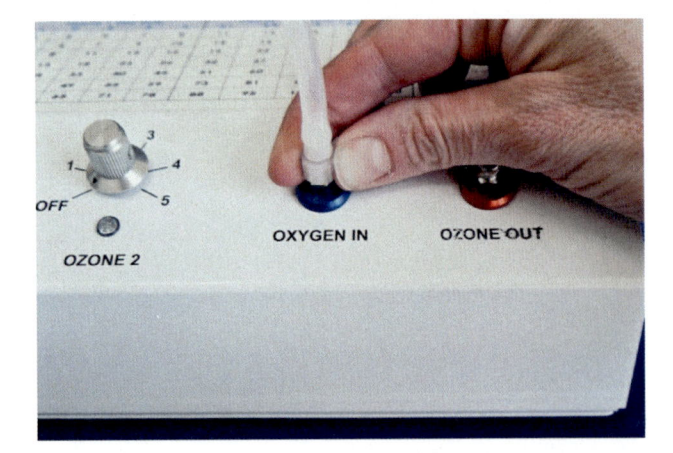

Step 7.3.7.
Screw the male luer lock connector with the silicone tubing into the "oxygen in" port of the ozone generator.

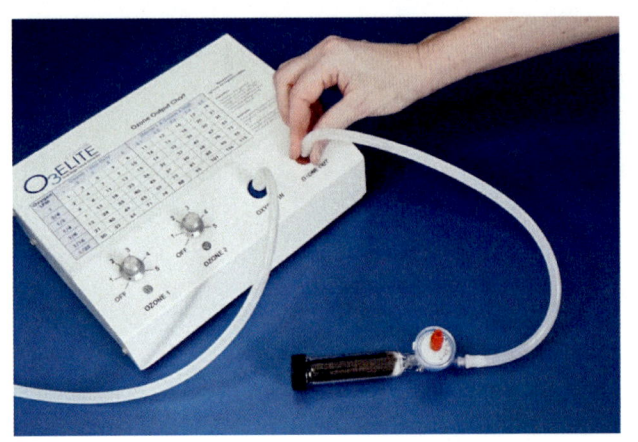

Step 7.3.8.
Connect the syringe filling station to the "ozone out" port by screwing the silicone tubing into the port.

Chapter 7 questions

1. List the two main tools which are used to create an air-tight oxygen circuit.
2. What can happen when silicone tubing is left on luer locks for too long?
3. Why should you not use PVC tubing for the oxygen path?

8. How to handle an oxygen tank

An oxygen tank contains gas under extreme pressure (200 to 300 bar). If a tank is mishandled, it could turn into a missile and do great damage to people and property. For this reason it is important to store oxygen tanks safely and handle them properly. Here is how:

8.1. Fixate it

An oxygen tank should be physically secured in a way that it cannot topple over. Either put it in a cart, bolt it to the wall with chains, or bind it to a sturdy table.

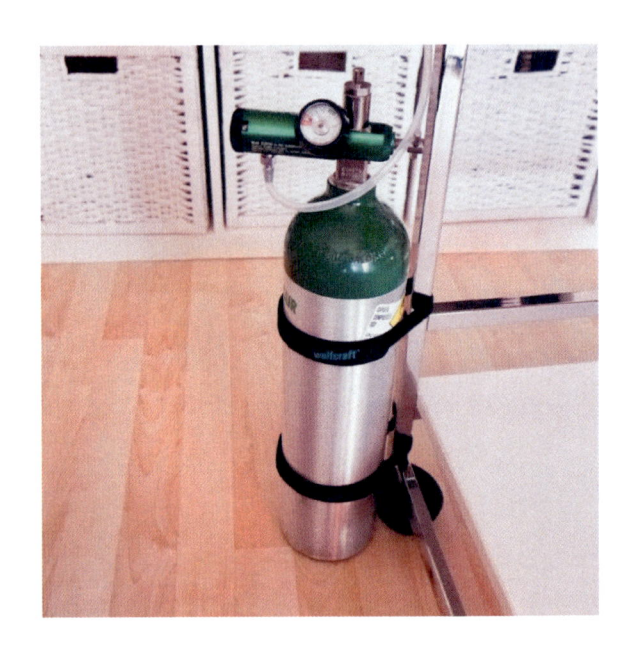

8.2. Keep away from heat

When a tank is exposed to high heat, the gas inside will expand which can make the valve burst. Do NOT keep a tank in the sun, close to a heater, or a stove.

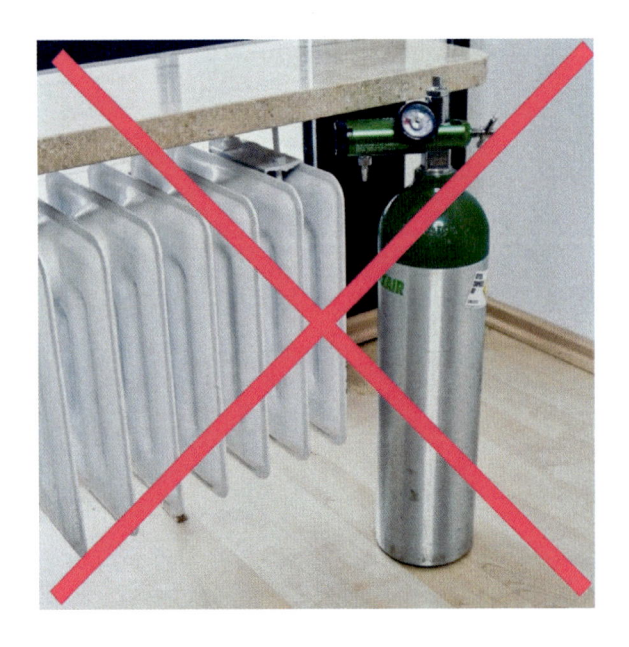

8.3. Keep away from oils

Do NOT apply any oils on the valve or the regulator of the tank since oxygen can increase combustibility.

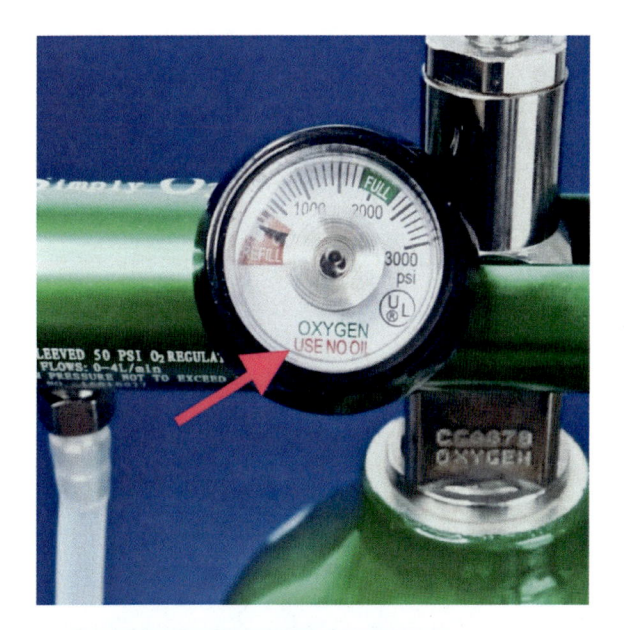

8.4. Half a turn to open

Open the tank with half a turn of the valve. That's enough. There is no need to open it all the way.

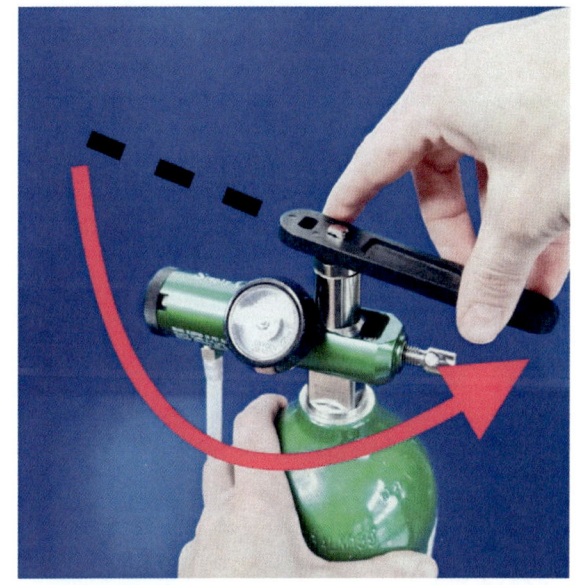

The same applies to an oxygen tank with a CGA 540 valve. Half a turn gets the job done.

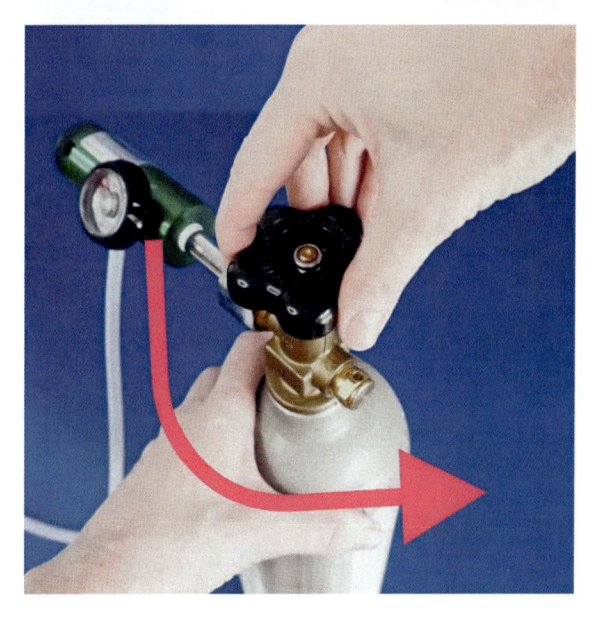

45

8.5. Do not exert too much pressure

When you close the tank, do not exert too much pressure: neither on the valve nor on the regulator. Closing the valve with too much force can damage the rubber seal and over time create a leak.

8.6. Inspection every 5 years

Tanks need to be inspected every 5 years, same for regulators. If the tank is older than 5 years, either get a new one or have it inspected by a local gas supplier. The oxygen itself does not go bad, but the valve can become compromised.

8.7. Get a wrench

If the tank has a straight post valve, don't forget to get a special wrench to open it.

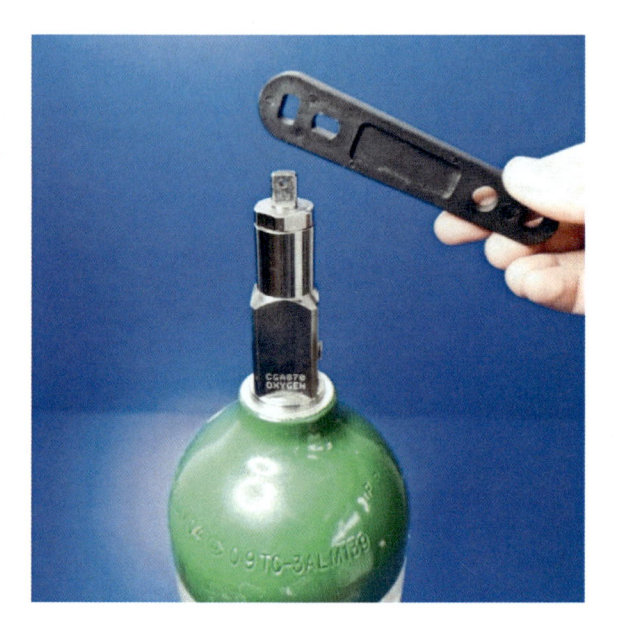

8.8. How to purge the regulator

To protect the regulator, It's important to release the pressure after each use. Do this after the 30 minute rest period.

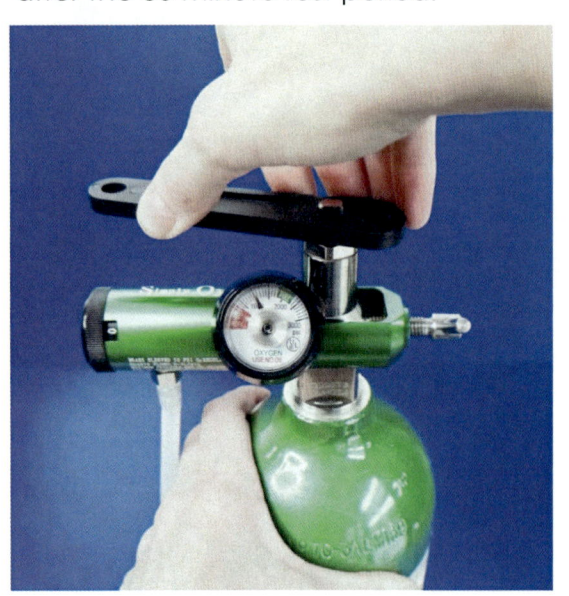

Step 8.8.1.

First, close the valve. Close it tightly, without exerting too much force.

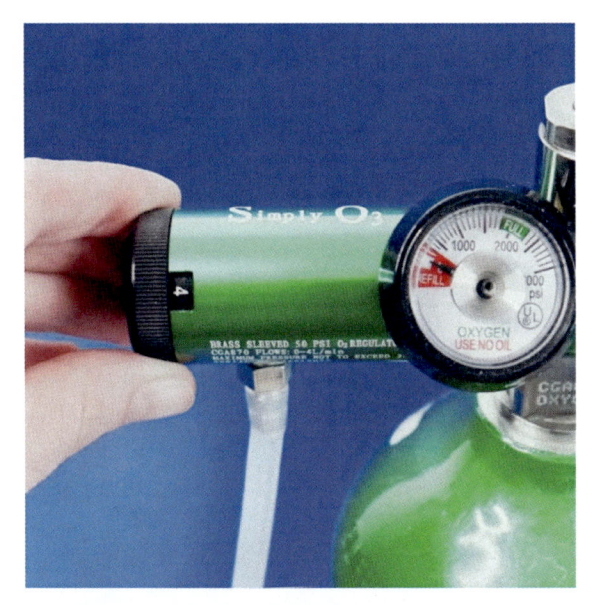

Step 8.8.2.
Open the regulator to the maximum flow. Watch the gauge as it goes down to zero. There will be a hissing sound.

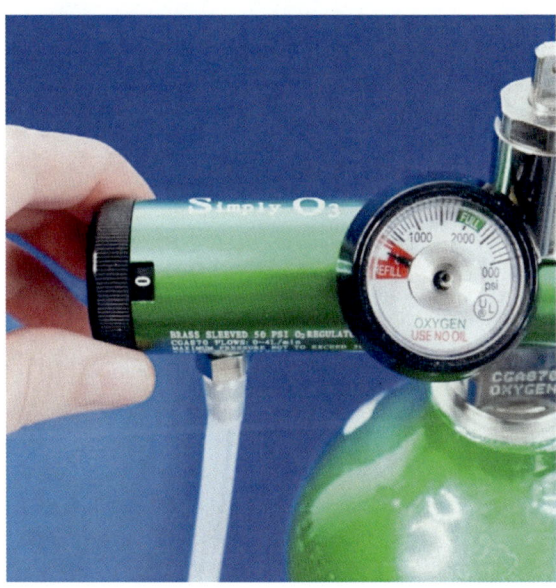

Step 8.8.3.
Once the gauge is all the way down, set the regulator to zero.

Chapter 8 questions

1. Why do oxygen tanks require special attention?
2. What is the correct way to open and close a tank?
3. Why should a tank be kept out of the sun?

Sources

[1] Intermountain Healthcare: "Portable Oxygen Cylinders Training and Safety Guidelines"
[2] Safety and Health Magazine: "Handling and storing compressed gas cylinders"
[3] Oxygo.life: "16 Tips for Oxygen Safety at Home"

9. Veins

Without finding a vein to inject, it's impossible to perform DIV ozone treatments. Understanding veins, how they run, how they need to be injected, and how to keep them healthy is consequently a crucial part of the DIV process.

9.1. Which veins can be injected?

In general, any visible vein can be used. This can be any vein on the arms, wrists, legs, or feet. The bigger and more pronounced the vein is, the more easily it can be injected and the less likely it will become inflamed.

A vein should be always injected **with** the blood flow, so in the direction of the heart.

Some veins can seem uncomplicated, but are actually more difficult to puncture like the veins on the wrists, which although often plump and well visible, are almost always so-called "rolling veins". When a needle is applied to them, they will move and make it very difficult to inject. Rolling veins have to be stabilized.

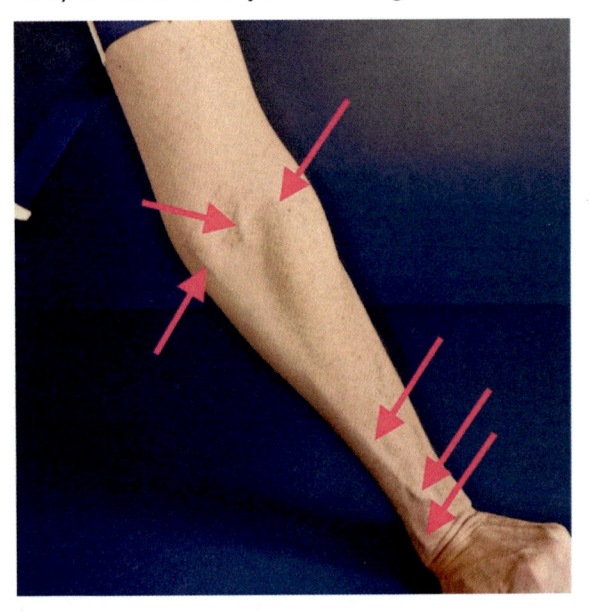

The most common vein to inject is the median cubital vein in the elbow pit (antecubital fossa). Other veins include branches of the cephalic and basilic veins. Veins around the wrist tend to be rolling veins which require being held in place or stretching to inject.

The great saphenous vein is located on the inside of the thighs and can be also used for DIV injections. When no other vein can be accessed, even veins on the foot can be used.

Varicose veins can be punctured as well, see chapter 12. Injecting varicose veins has several benefits: the bulging and discoloration of the vein can be eliminated and there is less risk of developing chest tightness.

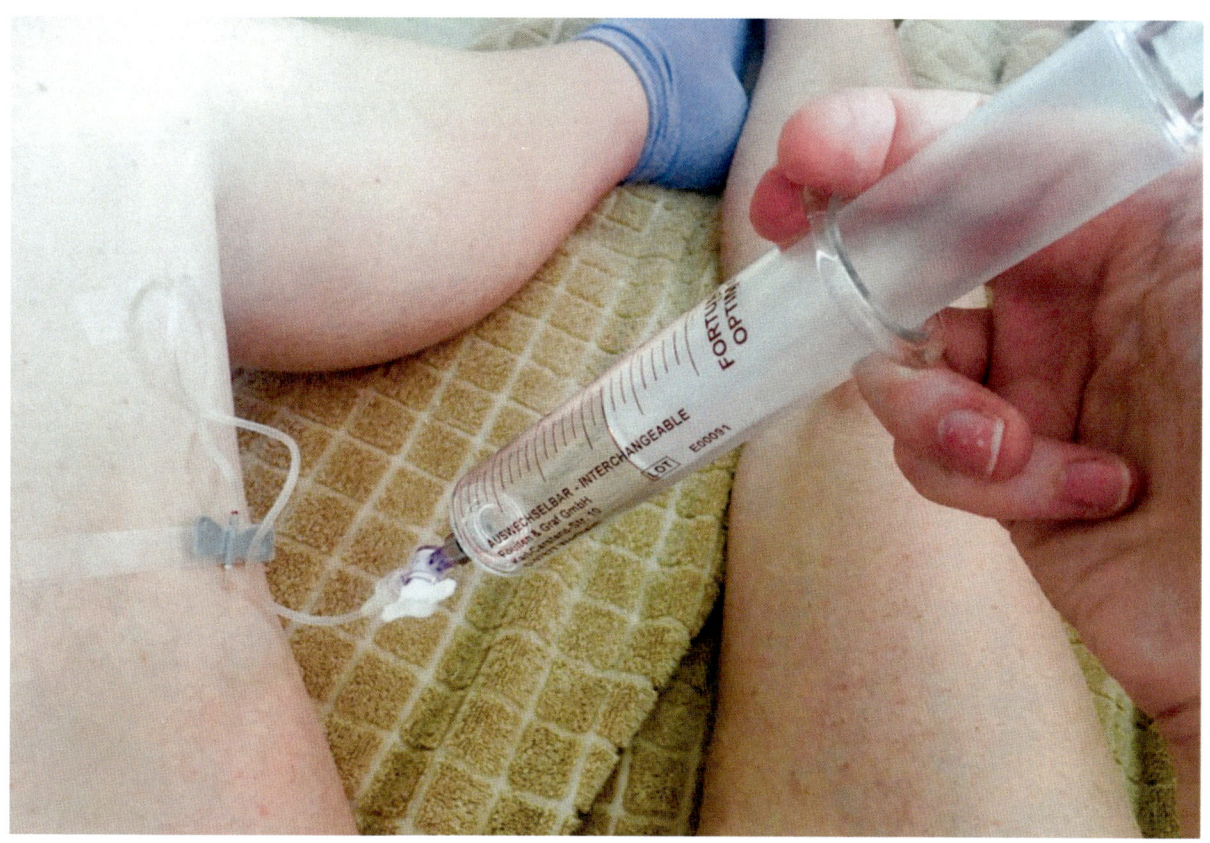

A DIV injection with a glass syringe into the great saphenous vein on the inner thigh.

Do leg veins carry a higher risk of Deep Vein Thrombosis?

A few ozone doctors are of the opinion that injecting lower extremities (legs and feet) carries a greater risk of causing dangerous DVT than injecting higher extremities (arms and hands).

Although this assertion appears a few times in the literature, I could not find any studies which substantiated it. The increased risk of DVT after IV administration appears to primarily deal with intravenous administration of chemotherapy and catheters (not butterfly needles) with large diameters which are left in the patients' veins for a prolonged time.

I could not find evidence that the injection of lower extremity veins with small gauge butterfly needles to perform single intravenous administration of non-chemotherapy drugs leads to a higher incidence of DVT.

It's still possible that this is an observed real phenomenon in clinical practice without there being any formal studies on the topic. So, it may make sense to keep this possible risk in mind. If you come across a study about DVT and injections of lower extremities, I would love to read it. Please, forward it to paola@thepowerofozone.com.

9.2. How to inject a vein

The injection of the vein is a four steps process: puncture, checking for blood, flattening, and pushing the needle in. With time this becomes one fluid movement.

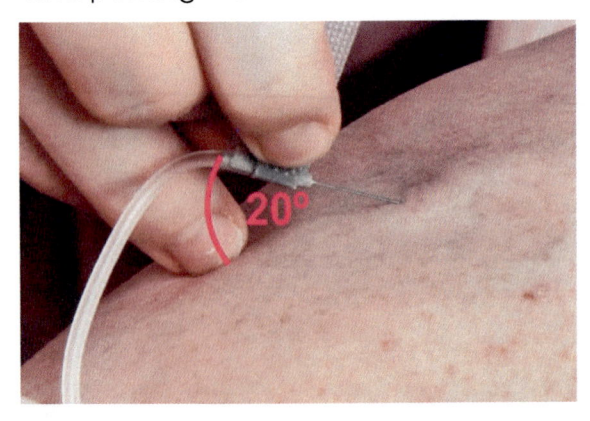

Puncture the vein: keep the needle at around a 15 to 20 degrees angle.

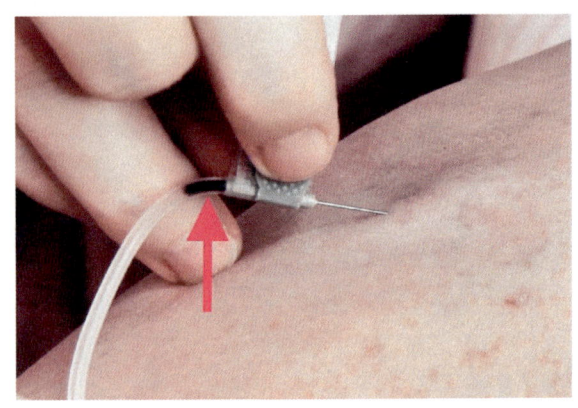

Check for blood backflow in the butterfly line. Do NOT proceed if there is no blood.

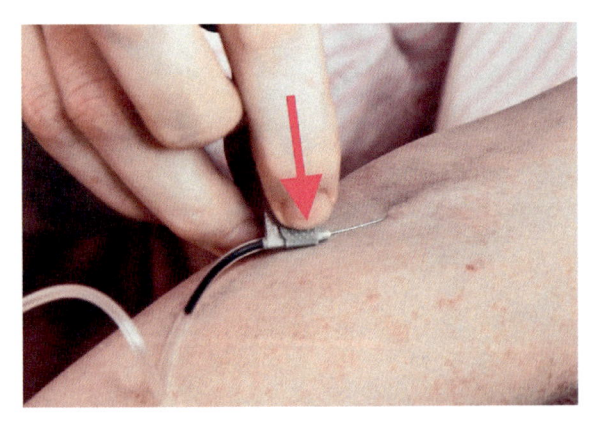

Flatten the needle against the skin.

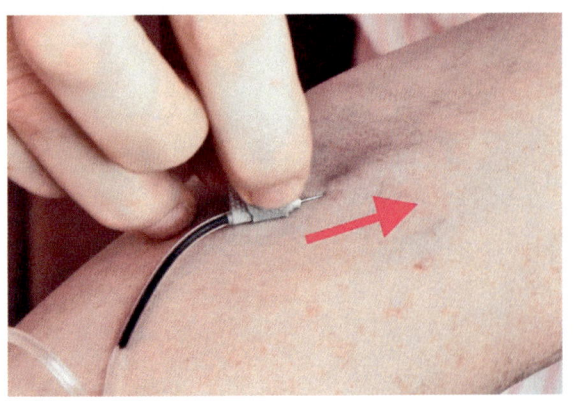

Push the needle in. The deeper it is placed, the more secure it is. Make sure you have the angle of the needle right, before you push it in, otherwise you'll puncture through the vein.

9.3. How to inject a rolling vein

Moving or rolling veins are those which move or roll when they are injected. Plump looking veins on wrists and feet are often deceiving: they look big and pronounced, but are often difficult to inject since they tend to move or roll when punctured. In order to successfully inject such a vein, it needs to be stabilized. Here's how:

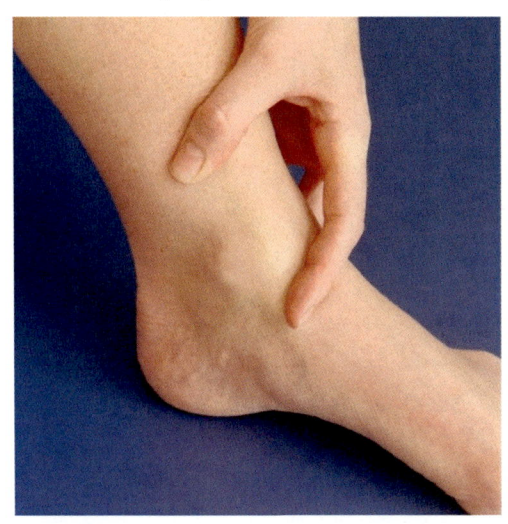

Use the index finger and the thumb to **stretch a vein** before the puncture. This can make the vein flatter, so it may be necessary to reduce the angle between needle and skin.

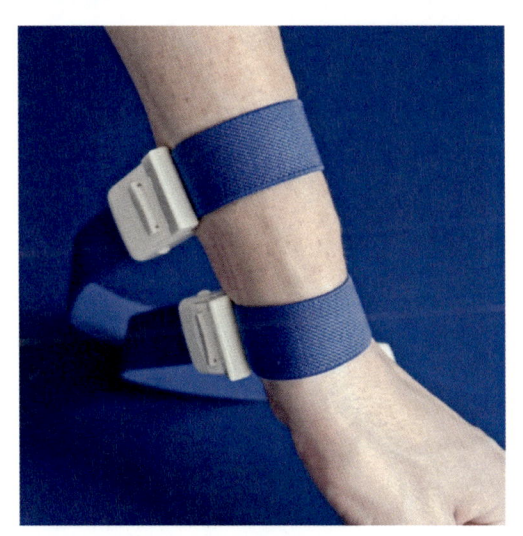

Another trick: Hold the vein in place between **two tourniquets** positioned closely to each other.

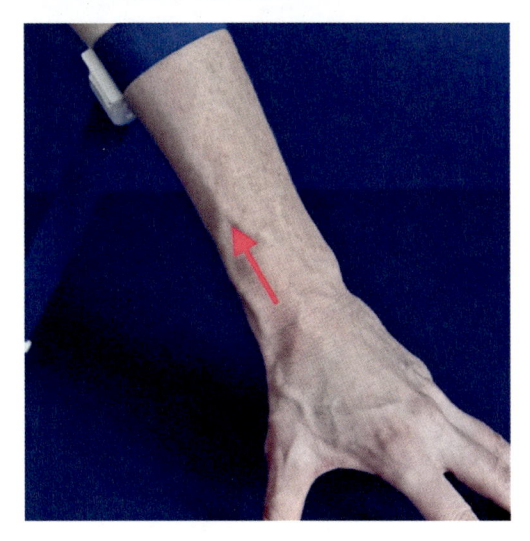

Find a Y-junction: this is a spot where two veins merge into one bigger vein. Inject into the merging point.

9.4. How to prevent and treat phlebitis

Phlebitis is the occurrence of inflammation of the vein and it is quite common with DIV ozone injections. Symptoms of phlebitis are redness, itchiness, swelling, pain, and hardening of the vein.

Repeated vein inflammation can create scar tissue which can make it very difficult or impossible to inject the vein in the future. To keep veins healthy, it's important to prevent inflammation as much as possible. Here are some suggestions how to achieve this:

Rotate veins
Use a different vein each time, especially if the injections are performed daily. This will allow the vein to recover from the previous puncture.

Use low ozone concentrations
Ozone concentrations between 20 and 35 mcg/ml are sufficient to achieve therapeutic effect. Higher amounts are not necessary, but increase the risk of phlebitis.

Load up on vitamin C
Start taking vitamin C before a DIV injection. The antioxidant will counteract some of the effect of the ozone and protect veins, but also diminish some of the therapeutic effect of the ozone therapy. So, be aware of the likely trade-off.

Ibuprofen or aspirin
Anti-inflammatory medication like ibuprofen or other NSAIDS right after or right before the DIV can both prevent and treat phlebitis.

Inject saline right after the DIV
Injecting 10 to 20 ml of 0.9% physiological saline right after the ozone treatment could lessen the inflammation.

Wait
Once phlebitis has occurred, it will resolve by itself after a while. This can be anything from a few hours to a few days. Just be patient!

Apply vitamin C and E
Apply a cream which contains vitamins C and/or E. The antioxidants will penetrate the skin and soothe the inflamed tissue.

Infrared light
Something which has been suggested by a member of our ozone community: apply infrared light. It's supposed to stimulate collagen production and so contribute to healing.

Proteolytic enzymes
Bromelain, serraptase, and nattokinase are enzymes which are recommended to prevent and treat sclerosed veins.

Arnica cream
Many people swear by this plant extract to help with any type of topical inflammatory signs. There is a wide range of arnica based creams to try out.

DMSO
Applying a light DMSO solution is another possible topical anti-inflammatory application.

Glutathione IVs
Especially as an IV or push right after the DIV, glutathione will prevent an irritation of the vein. But it will also diminish ozone's therapeutic effect.

WARNING: *Glutathione has been reported to create devastating effects in many people, including the sensation of rods in the skull, crushing fatigue, debilitating headaches, neuropathy, and an often reported "feeling like dying". Which is why I do not recommend them, but some people seem to do fine with it and may want to take the risk to protect their veins.*

9.5. How to make veins visible
Sometimes veins are not well visible, or they are small and hidden which makes them difficult to inject. Here is a collection of tips and tricks on how to make veins plump up:

- **Drink**

Make sure you're well hydrated. Drink 1 to 2 big glasses of water before an injection.

- **Slap it**

Slap the vein. This increases the circulation and makes the vein become more prominent.

- **Apply warmth**

Pour warm water or put a warm washcloth over the injection site.

- **Use the "touch the ground" trick**

I learned this when I worked at a doctor's office. The doctor would have a very pronounced tremor in his hands and yet he would always find a vein. If neither me nor any of my co-workers had luck in puncturing a patient, as a last resort we would send the patient to the doctor knowing that he would always succeed. I asked him what the trick was. Here is what he taught me:

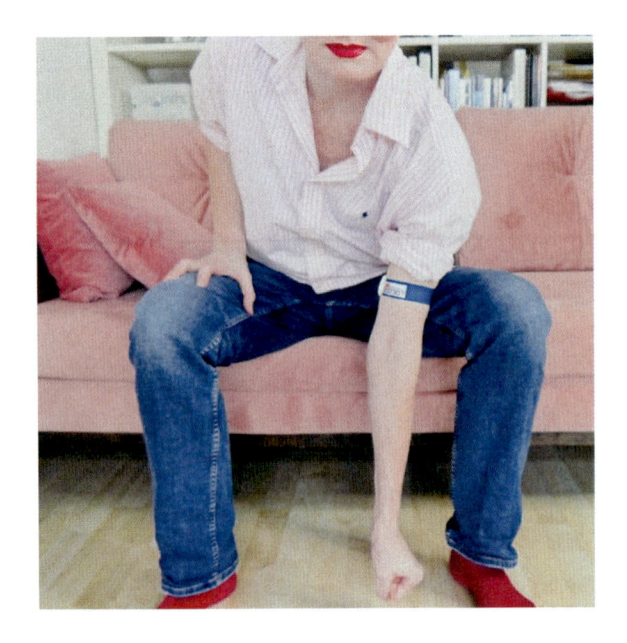

Ask the patient to lower the arm all the way to the ground and keep pumping the fist.

Apply the tourniquet and watch how the vein fills up and becomes easy to inject.

Chapter 9 questions

1. Can varicose veins be used to perform DIV ozone injections?
2. Which direction should the needle point to when injecting a vein?
3. What is the problem with veins around the wrist?
4. Explain two ways to inject a rolling vein.
5. What is the best trick to make difficult veins more visible?

Sources
[1] Vascular Medicine, angiologist.com: "Catheter Associated Thrombosis"
[2] Healthline.com: "Superficial Thrombophlebitis"
[3] Mount Sinai: "Superficial thrombophlebitis"
[4] Team Rapid Response: "Rapid Guide to IV Starts", 2015
[5] R. Scott Evans, et al: "Risk of symptomatic DVT associated with peripherally inserted central catheters"
[6] Arthur Steinberg: "The employment of the dimethyl sulfoxide as an antiinflammatory agent and steroid-transporter in diversified clinical diseases", 1967
[7] Deborah Penteado Martins Dias: "Jugular thrombophlebitis in horses: A review of fibrinolysis, thrombus formation, and clinical management", 2013

10. "DIV for the Superparanoid"

The "DIV for the Superparanoid" method is based on the following four principles:

1. **Ozone is heavier than air.**

2. **Never inject air into the vein, always pure oxygen/ozone mix.**

3. **The absorption of oxygen by the red blood cells is not always an instantaneous process. Depending on the individual, it can take a while for the gas to be taken up.**

4. **Gas rises in the human body to the highest point, the brain.**

Suggested ozone concentration: 20 to 35 mcg/ml. Suggested oxygen flow when filling the syringe is ½ LPM.

Step-by-step procedure

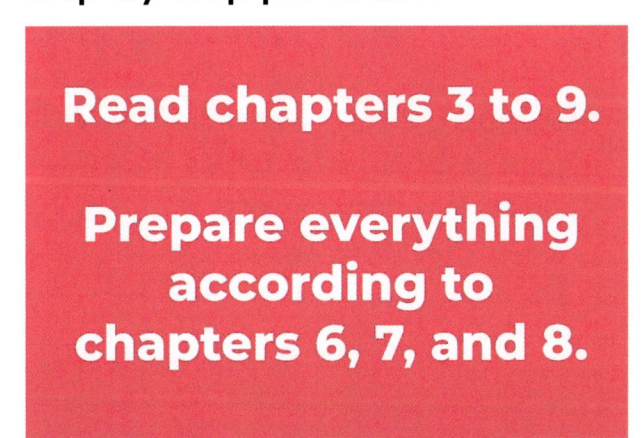

Step 10.1.
First, read chapters 1 to 9, and prepare everything according to instructions in chapters 6, 7, and 8.

Make sure to familiarize yourself with the syringe filling station.

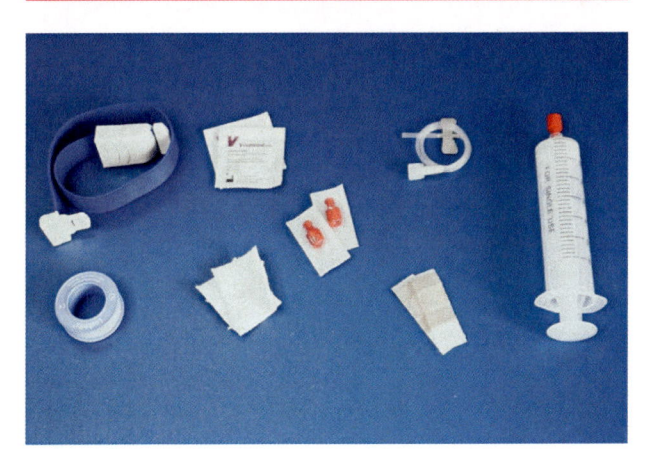

Step 10.2.
Prepare all the supplies: alcohol wipes, the butterfly needle, a tourniquet, cotton pads, a band-aid, syringe caps, and the syringe.

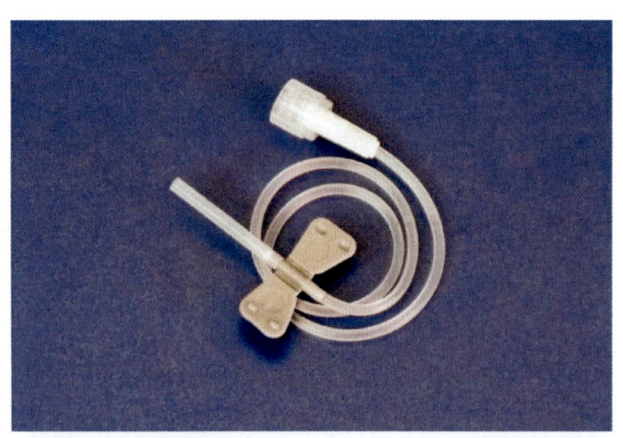

Step 10.3.
Make sure the butterfly needle is unwrapped. Leave the luer cap and the needle cap on.

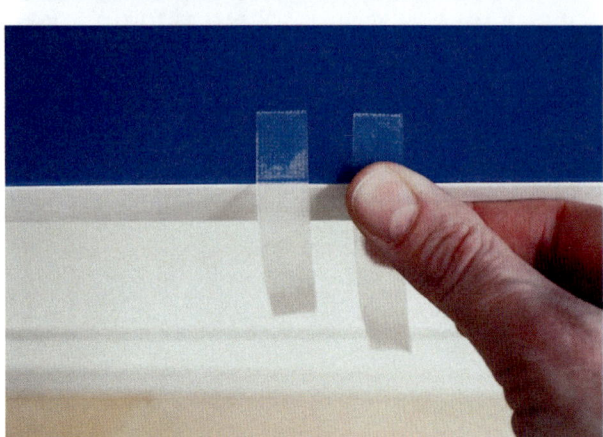

Step 10.4.
Prepare two pieces of tape, each around 3 inches long.

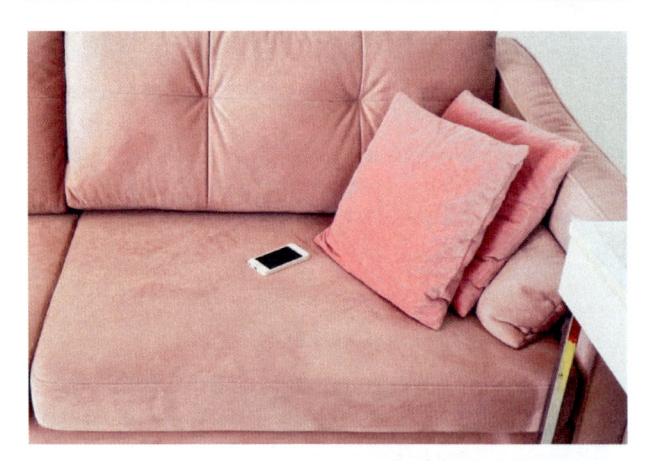

Step 10.5.
Place a book or a tablet on the couch or bed, where you will perform the injection.

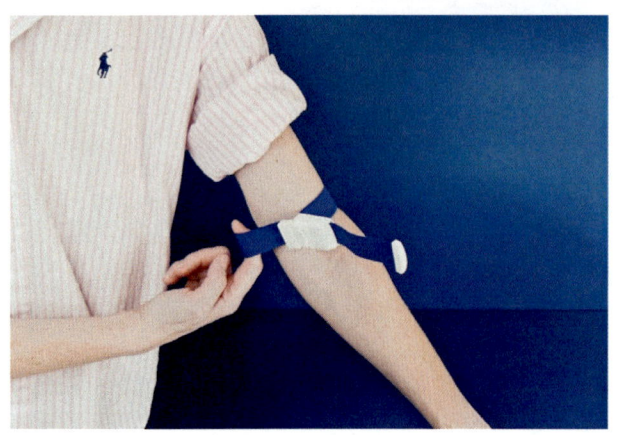

Step 10.6.
Put the tourniquet on your arm, loosely. Just park it there, do not tighten it.

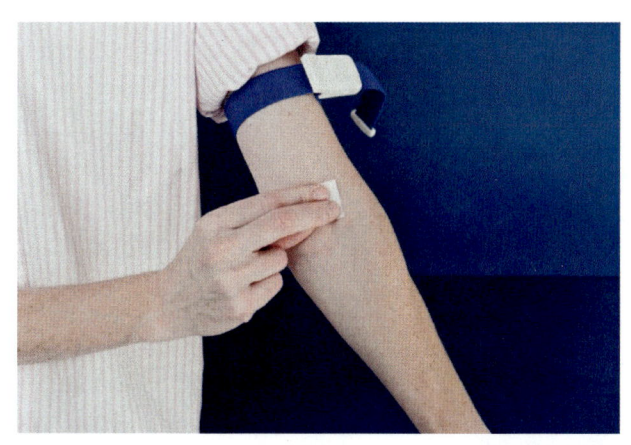

Step 10.7.
Take an alcohol wipe and disinfect the part of your arm where you will puncture the vein.

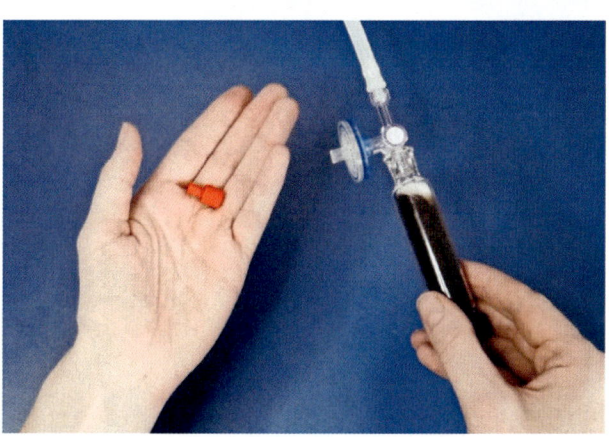

Step 10.8.
Remove the cap from the filter on the syringe filling station.

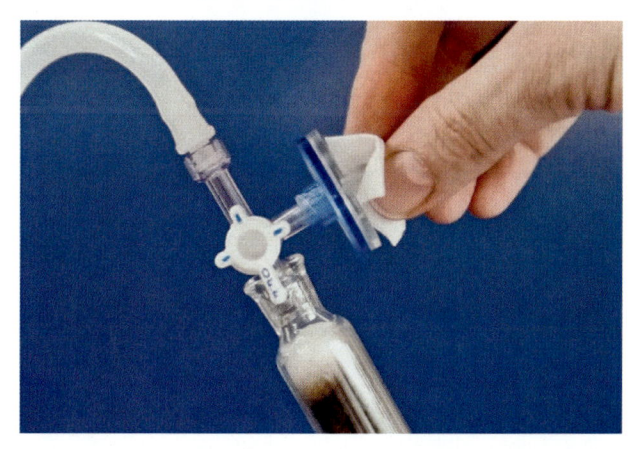

Step 10.9.
Wipe the opening of the filter with an alcohol wipe for 20 seconds.

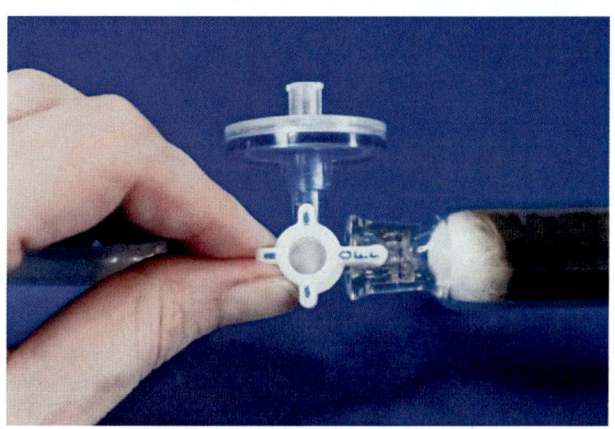

Step 10.10.
Make sure the OFF valve on the syringe filling station points towards the destructor.

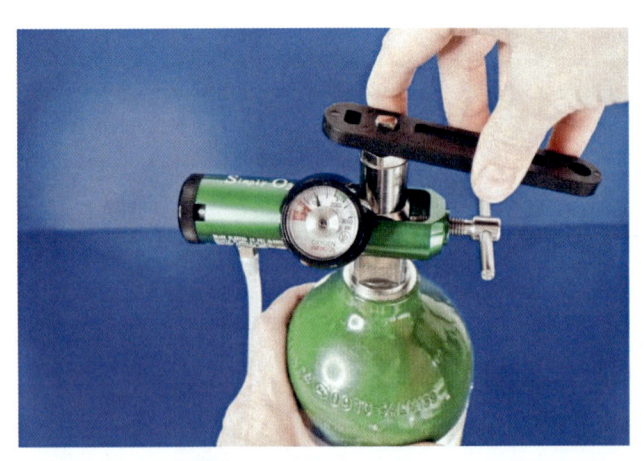

Step 10.11.
Open the valve of the tank using a wrench. Half a turn is enough. Watch the gauge on the regulator jump up. It shows if there is oxygen in the tank.

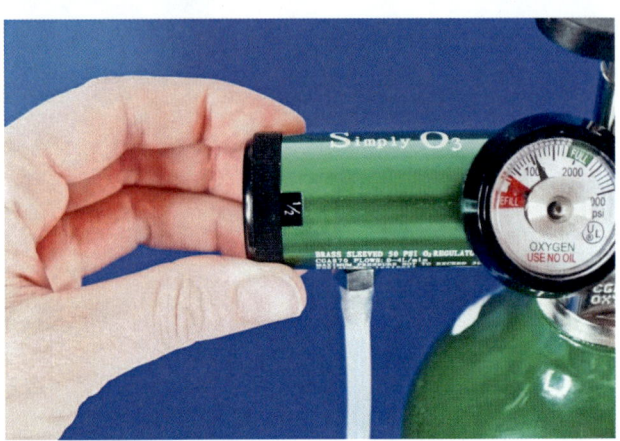

Step 10.12.
Open regulator to ½ LPM. You have now established an oxygen flow.

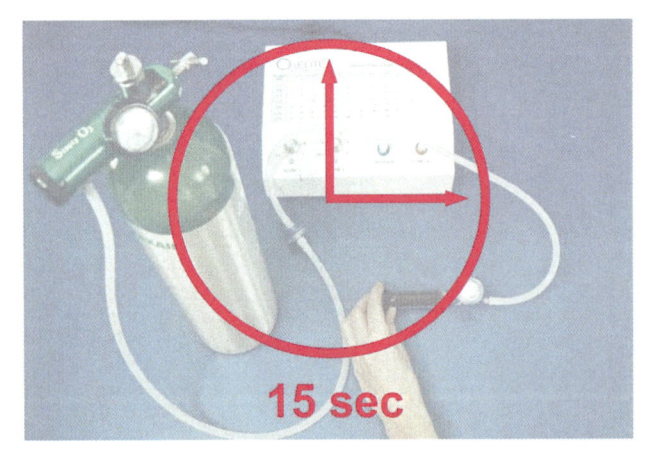

Step 10.13.
Let the oxygen run for 15 seconds to flush all the lines and saturate them with pure oxygen while keeping the filter pointing upwards.

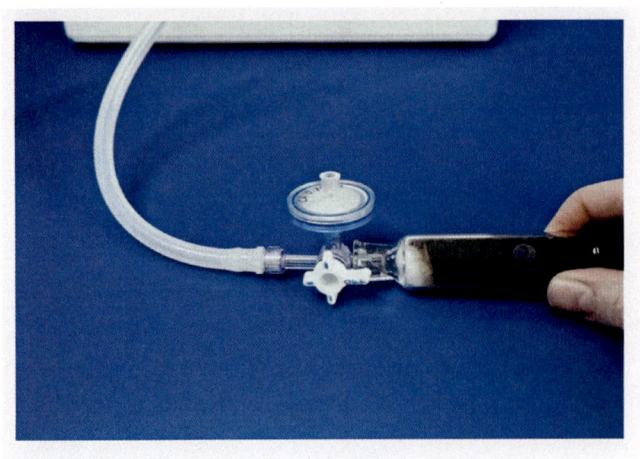

Closeup of step 10.13.
Keep the filter pointing up while oxygen flows through to make sure the gas stays in the filter and does not pour out allowing air to enter.

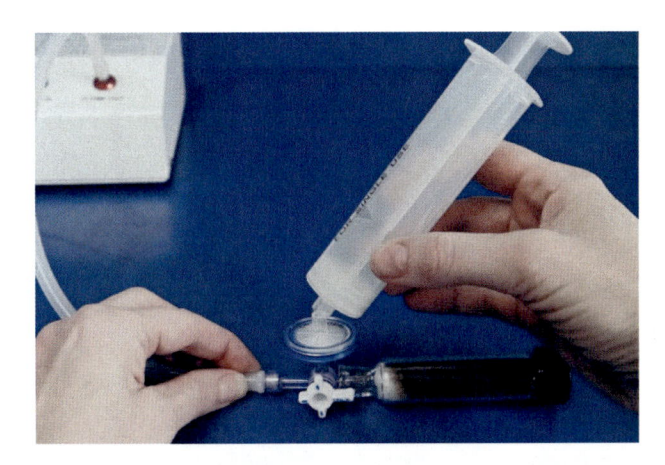

Step 10.14.
Now flush the syringe: attach it to the syringe filling station ...

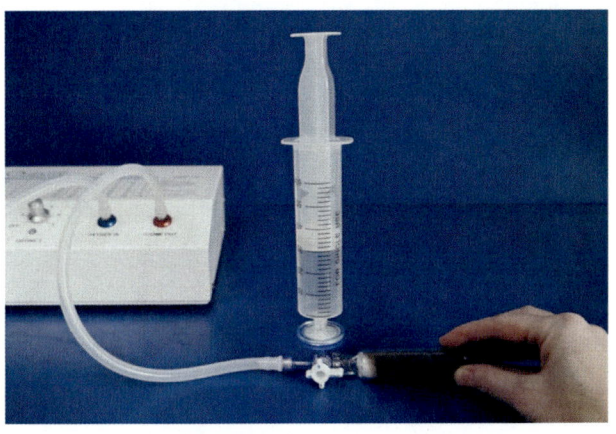

... and let it fill up.

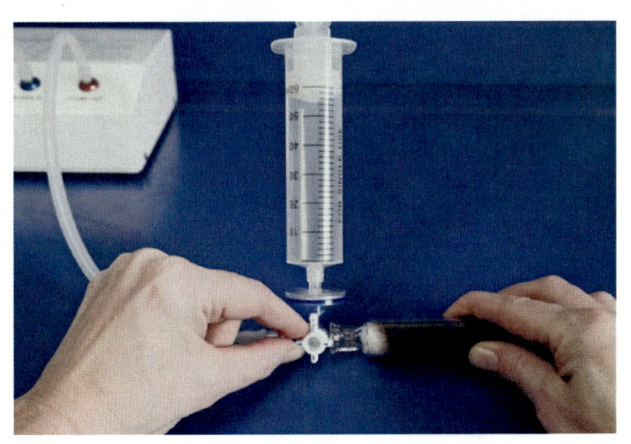

Step 10.15.
When full, close the syringe port by turning the OFF lever towards the syringe.

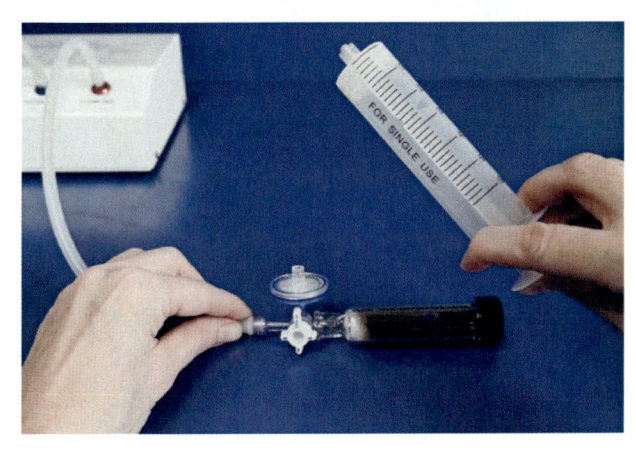

Step 10.16.
Unscrew the syringe and empty it while holding the syringe filling station upright the whole time.

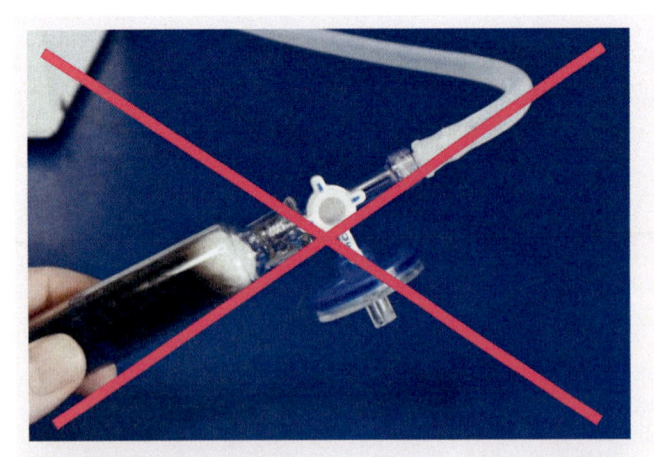

Explanation of steps 10.15. and 10.16.
It is important to keep the filter facing up when unscrewing the syringe, otherwise the oxygen could pour out and air could enter.

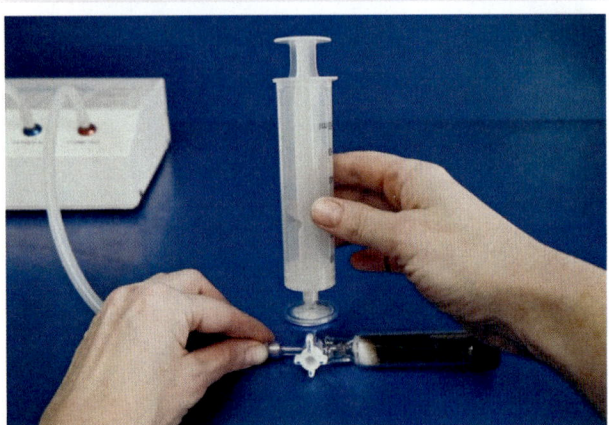

Step 10.17.
Screw the syringe onto the syringe filling station.

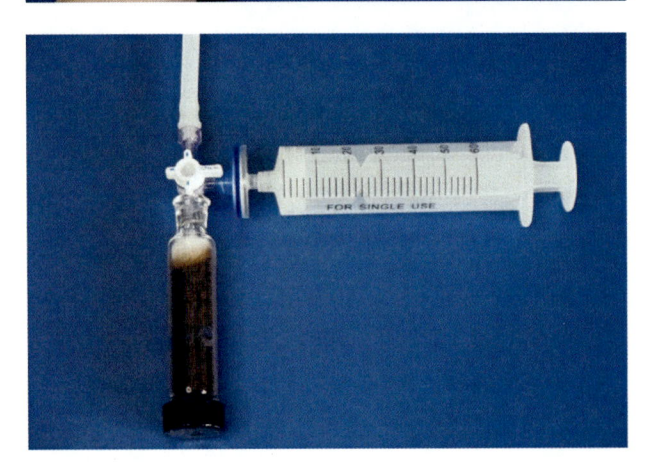

Step 10.18.
You can now let go of the filling station since you created a closed circuit.

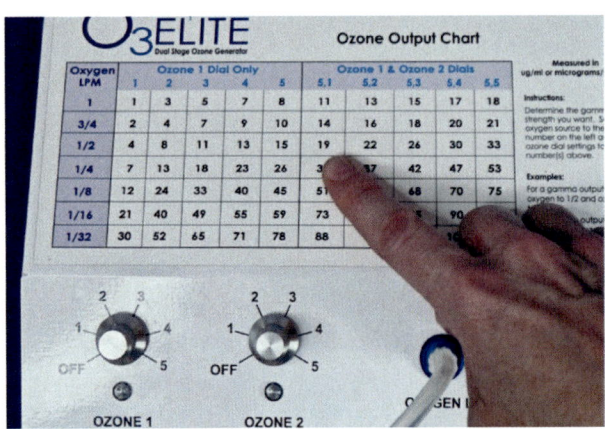

Step 10.19.
Choose the preferred ozone output on your generator. Keep the flow high at ½ LPM. Here, 19 mcg/ml are selected.

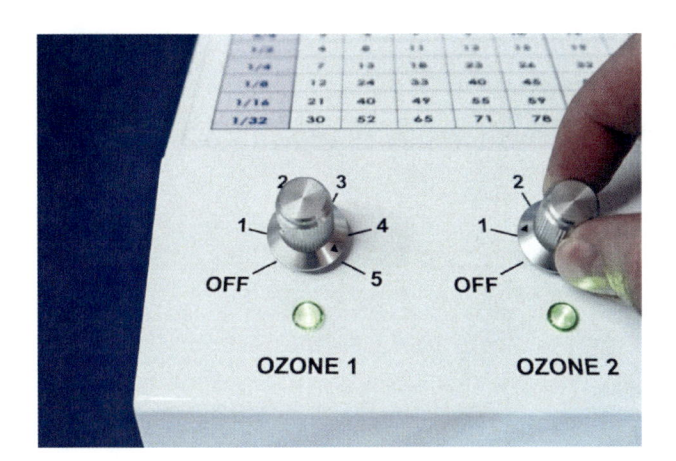

Step 10.20.
Turn the ozone generator on.

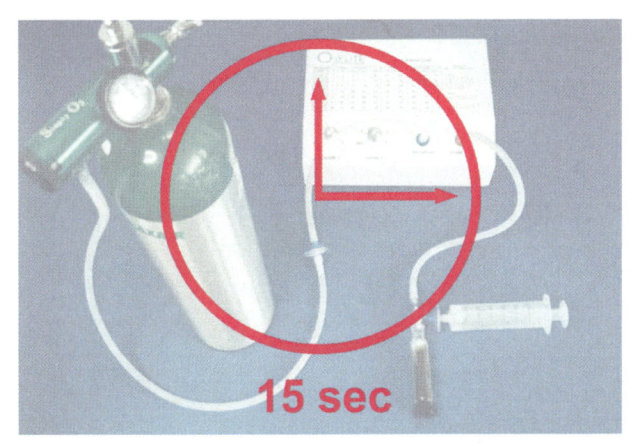

Step 10.21.
Wait 15 seconds for the ozone generator to start producing ozone.

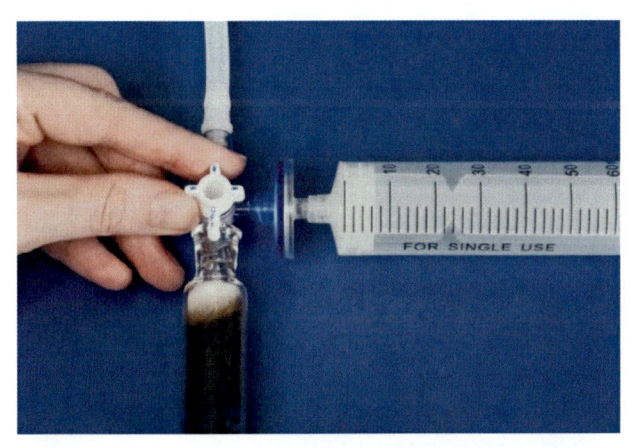

Step 10.22.
Open the port on the syringe filling station by turning the off valve toward the destructor.

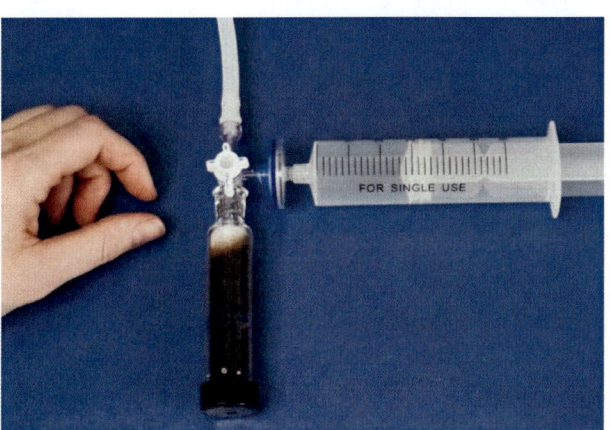

Step 10.23.
Fill the syringe. It will go fast, so keep your hand close by.

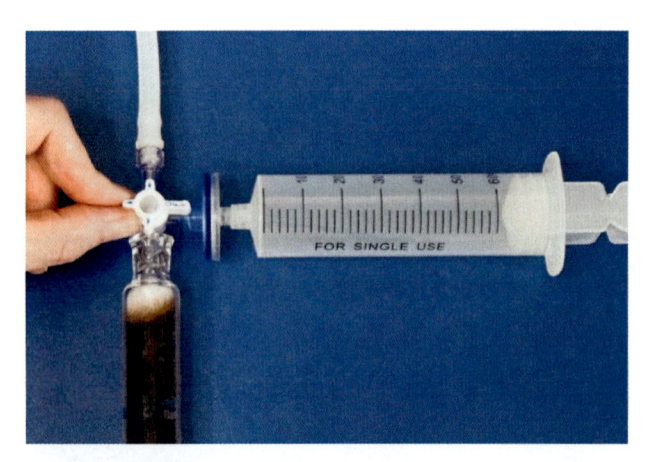

Step 10.24.

When the syringe is full, close the syringe port by turning the OFF lever towards the syringe.

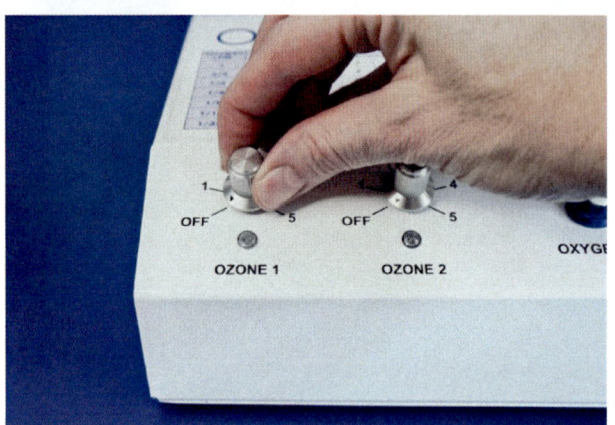

Step 10.25.

Turn the ozone generator off.

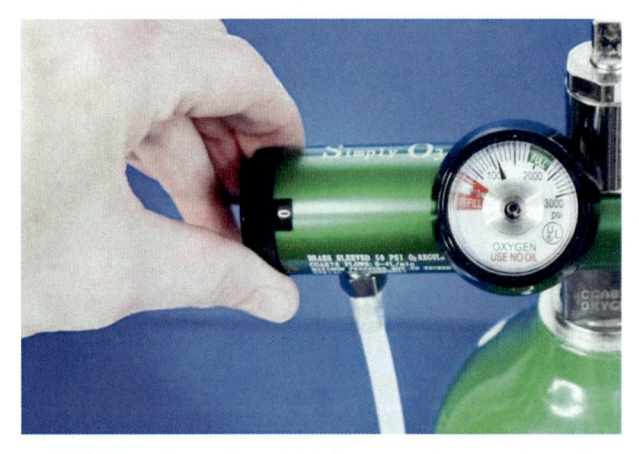

Step 10.26.

Turn the regulator to zero. Leave the valve open. You will take care of it later.

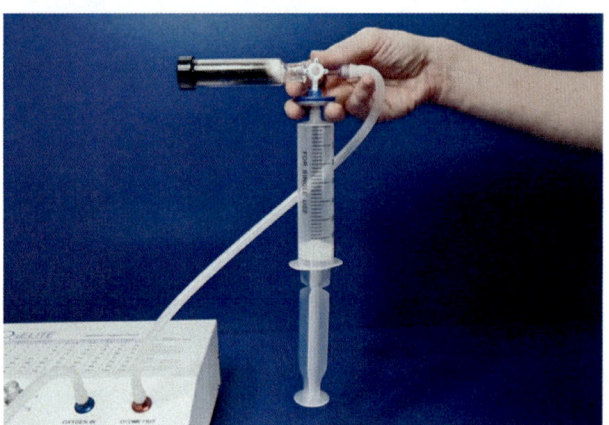

Step 10.27.

Hold the syringe filling station up (with the syringe attached to it), so that the syringe is vertical.

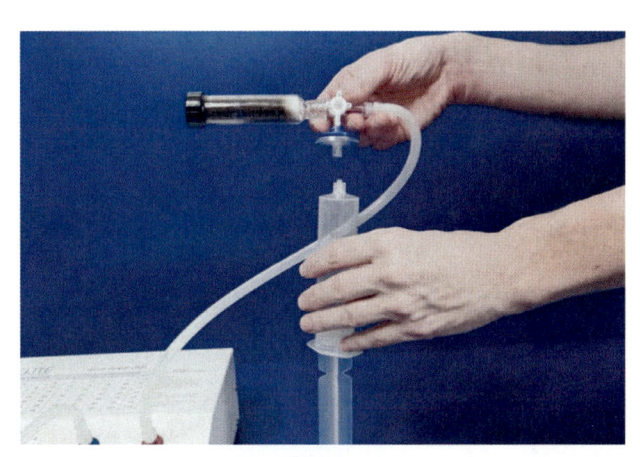

Step 10.28.

Unscrew the syringe. Keep the syringe vertically and the syringe opening pointing up at all times.

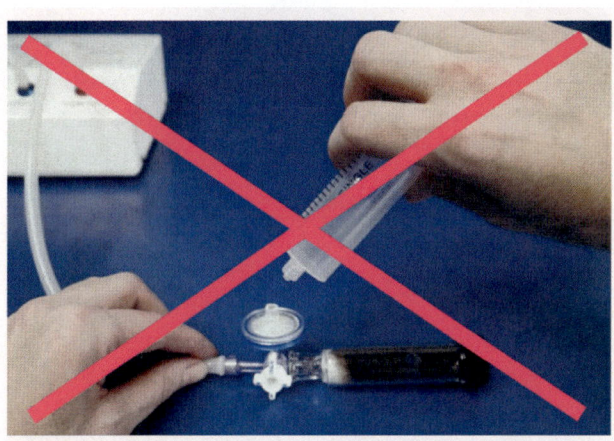

Explanation of steps 10.27. and 10.28.
If the syringe points down when it is unscrewed from the filling station, ozone/oxygen could pour out and air could enter. Don't ever flip the syringe.

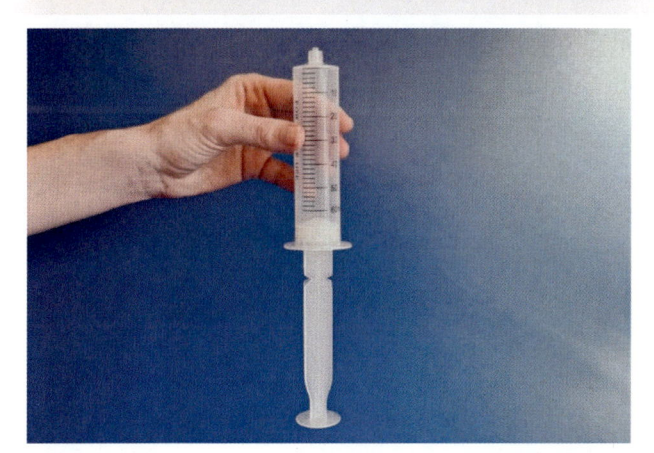

Step 10.29.

Do NOT flip it. Do not put it down. Do not lay it down. Hold it vertically the whole time.

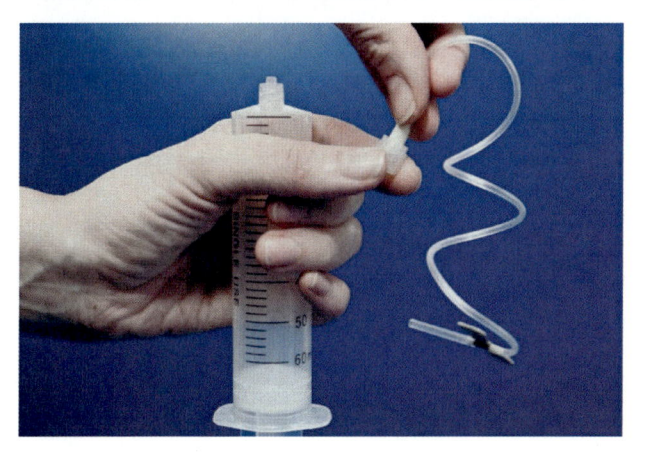

Step 10.30.

Take the butterfly needle and remove the cap from the end of the line. Keep the syringe vertical the whole time.

63

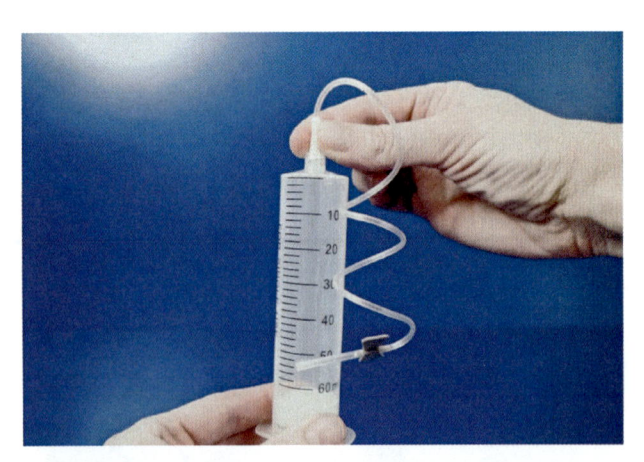

Step 10.31.
Screw the needle onto the syringe.

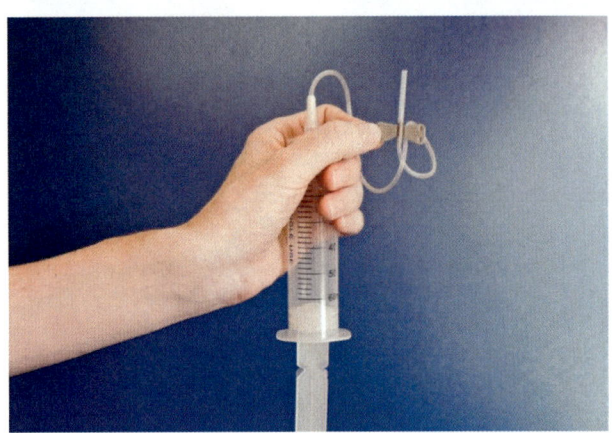

Step 10.32.
Hold the wings of the needle between index finger and thumb. Make sure that the needle is at the same level as the top of the syringe.

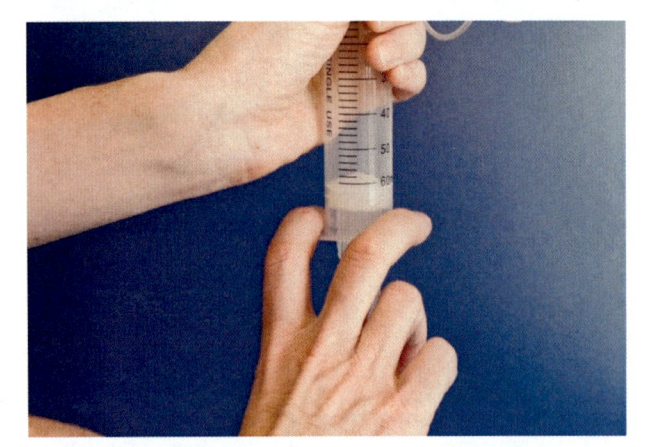

Step 10.33.
Flush the line of the butterfly needle: push out 5 cc. Keep the syringe upright at all times.

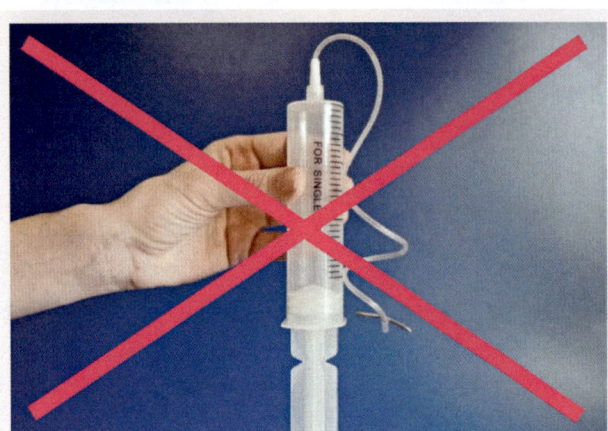

Explanation of steps 10.32. and 10.33.
Do not let the butterfly needle dangle after you have purged the line. Otherwise ozone, being heavier than air, could flow out and air could enter.

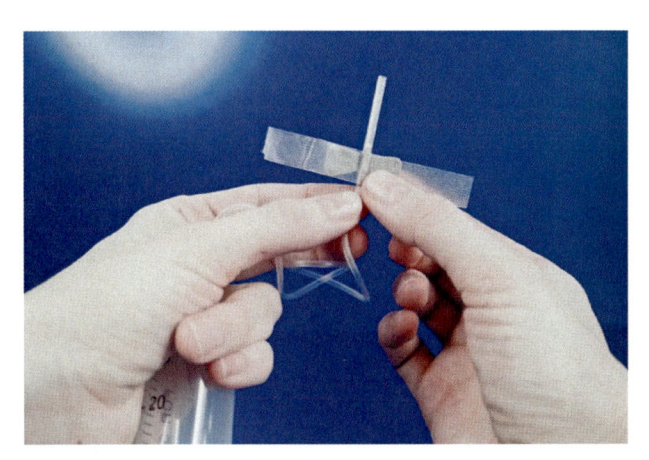

Step 10.34.
Take a piece of tape and tape it over the wings on the side with the ridge.

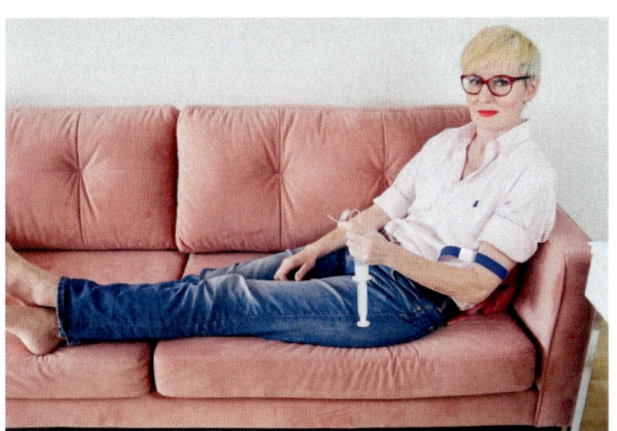

Step 10.35.
Move to where you will perform the injection. Place yourself in a reclined position. Keep holding the syringe vertically and the thumb and the index finger gripping the butterflies of the needle.

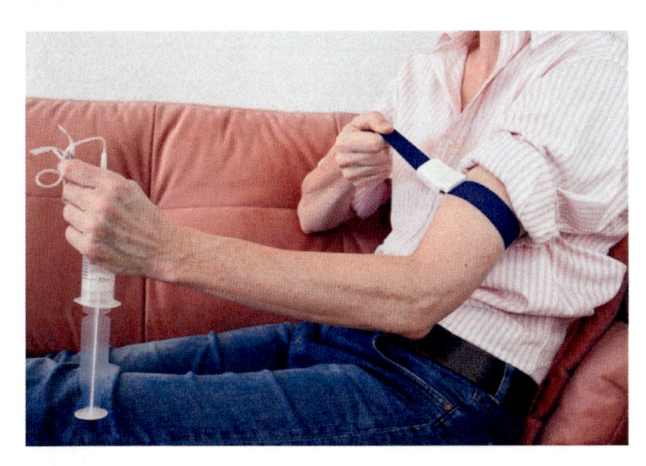

Step 10.36.
With your dominant hand, tighten the tourniquet. Keep holding the syringe vertically.

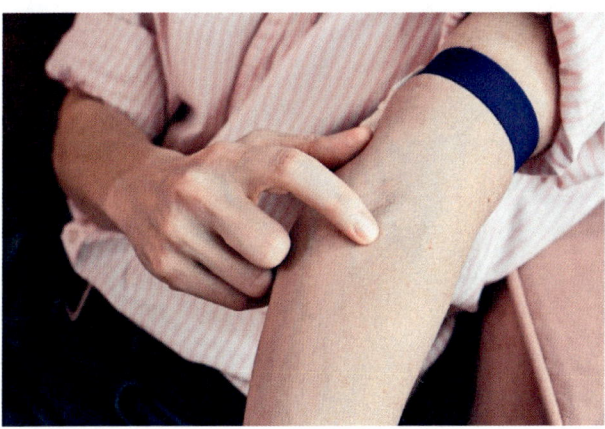

Step 10.37.
Wait for the vein to get plump and visible. Palpate it, get a feel for it, understand how it runs.

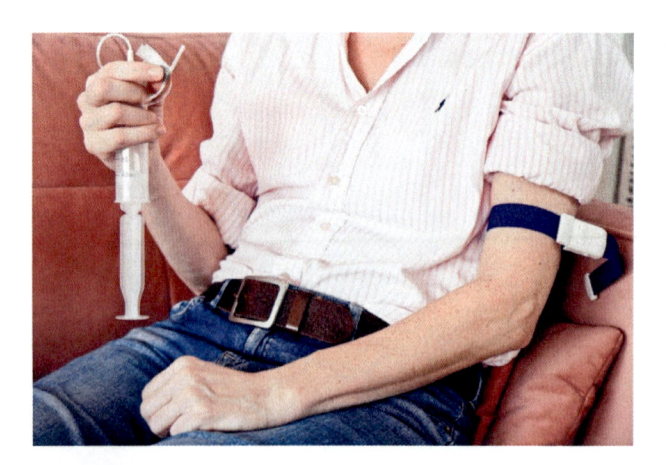

Step 10.38.
Switch the syringe and needle into your dominant hand.

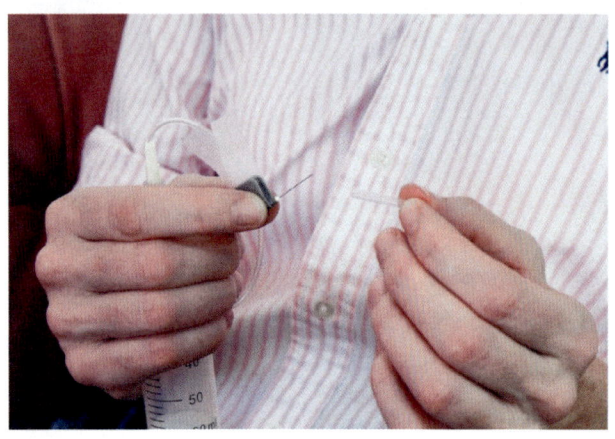

Step 10.39.
Remove the cap from the butterfly needle.

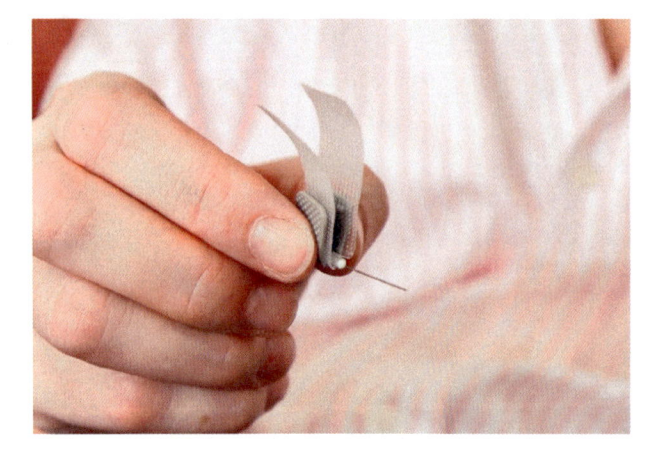

Step 10.40.
Grab the butterfly wings of the needle and pinch them between your index finger and thumb of your dominant hand.

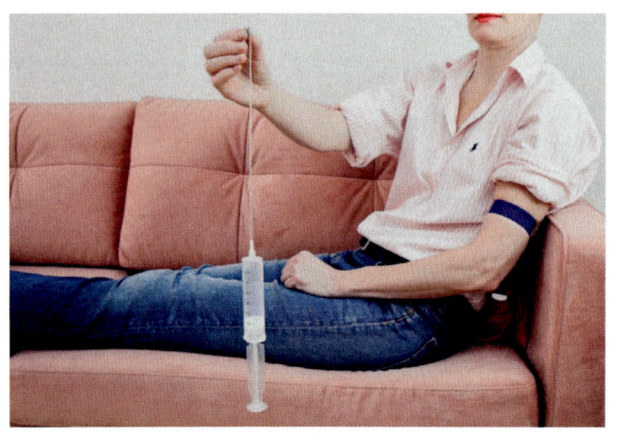

Step 10.41.
Let the syringe dangle to straighten out the line and to prepare to be grabbed by your non-dominant hand.

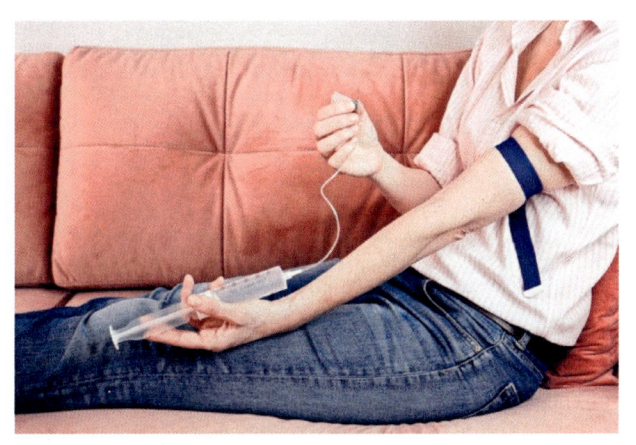

Step 10.42.
Hold the syringe as shown in the picture. Make sure that up to the point of injection the syringe is always positioned below the needle.

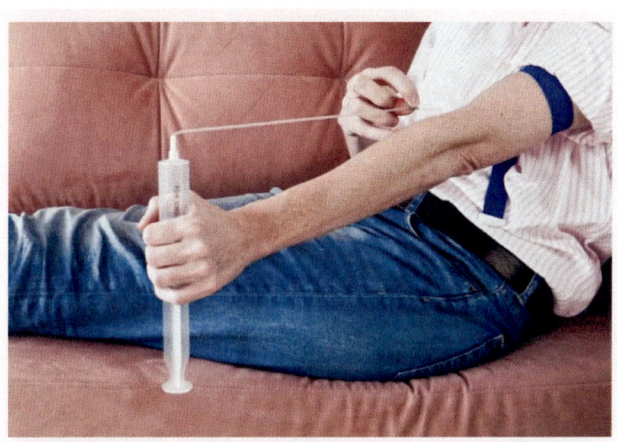

Explanation of step 10.42.
If you hold the syringe upright instead of laying it flat in your palm, you won't have enough slack in the tubing to be able to perform the injection.

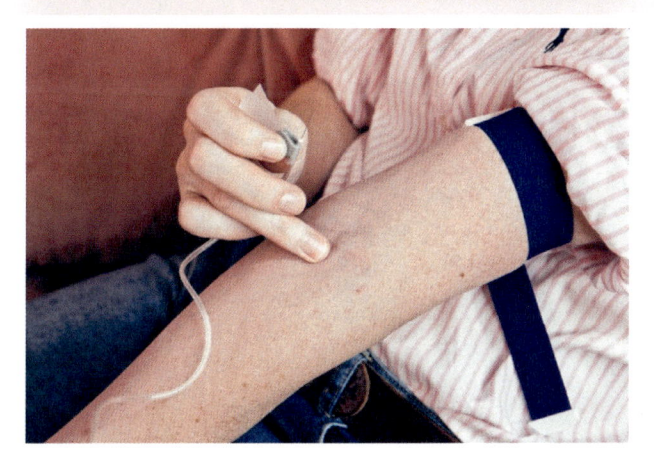

Step 10.43.
Palpate the vein again and understand in which angle it runs.

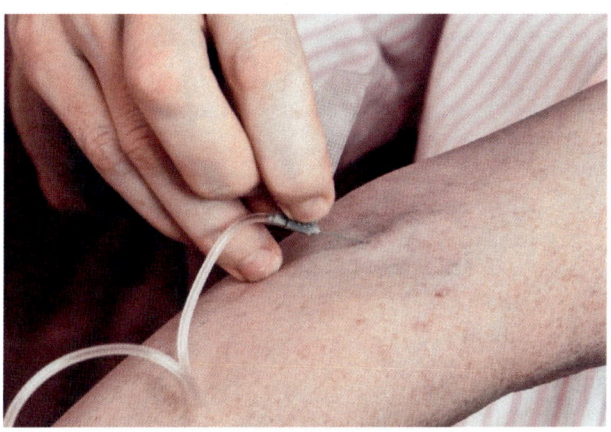

Step 10.44.
Hold the needle at a 15 to 20 degrees angle and puncture the vein.

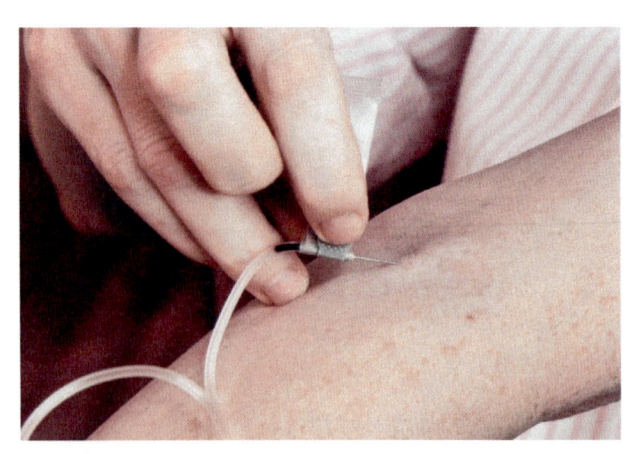

Step 10.45.
Check for blood in the line. If there is blood, it means you are in the vein and you can proceed with the next step. (If there is no blood, you are not in the vein and you need to adjust the needle or abort.)

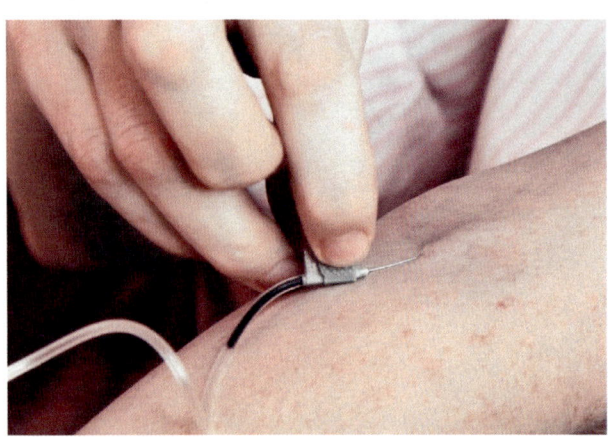

Step 10.46.
Flatten the needle against the skin.

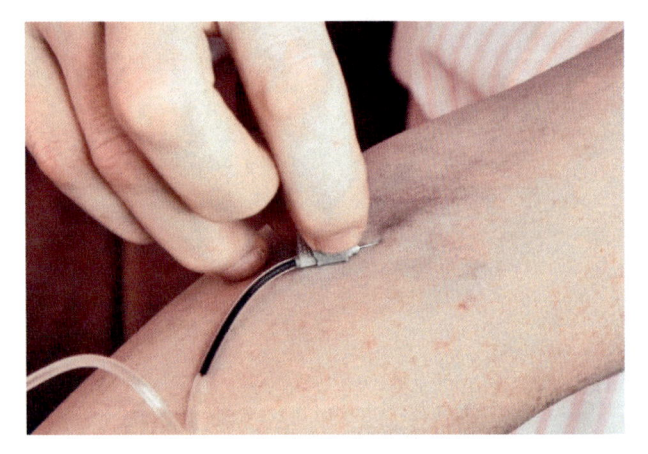

Step 10.47.
Push the needle into the vein. Most of the needle length should be inserted into the vein.

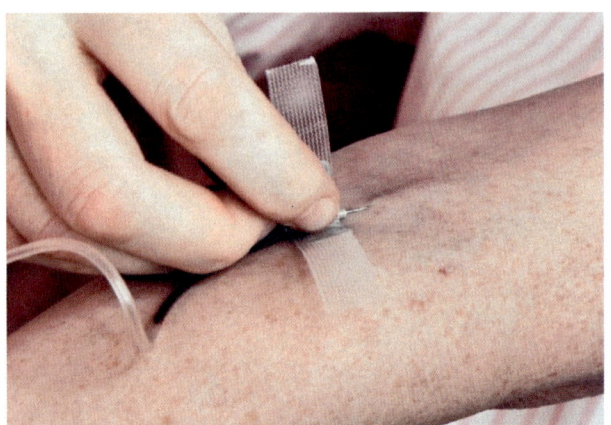

Step 10.48.
Spread the butterfly wings apart by releasing one wing and placing your index finger between them ...

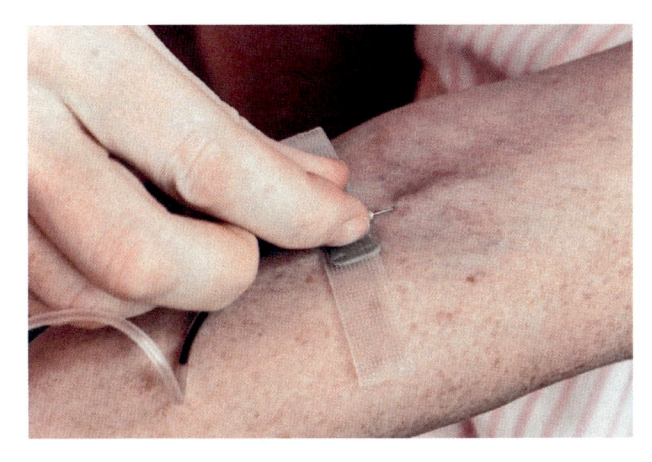

... and tape both butterfly wings down securely to your arm ...

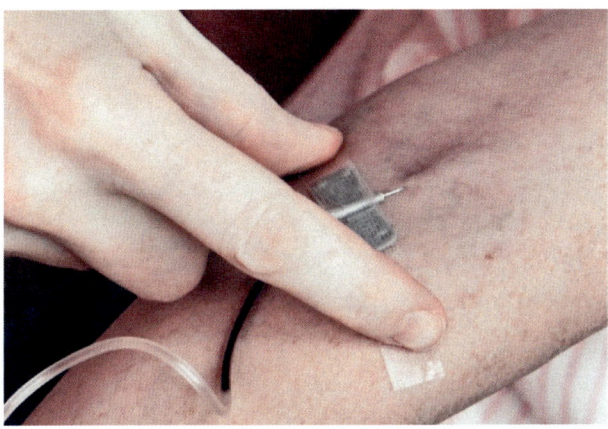

... with one movement.

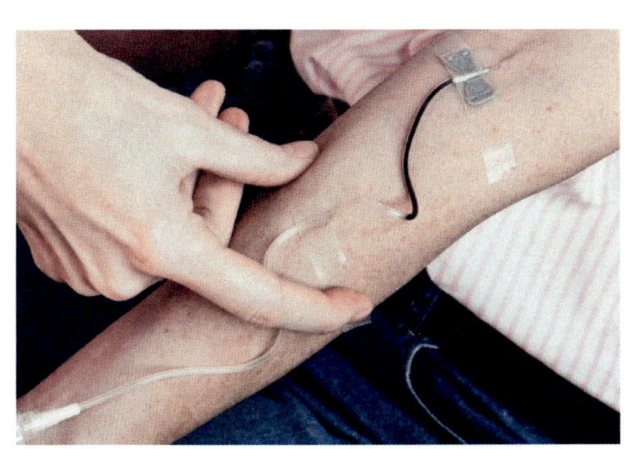

Step 10.49.
Take the other piece of tape and tape the line of the butterfly needle further down the line.

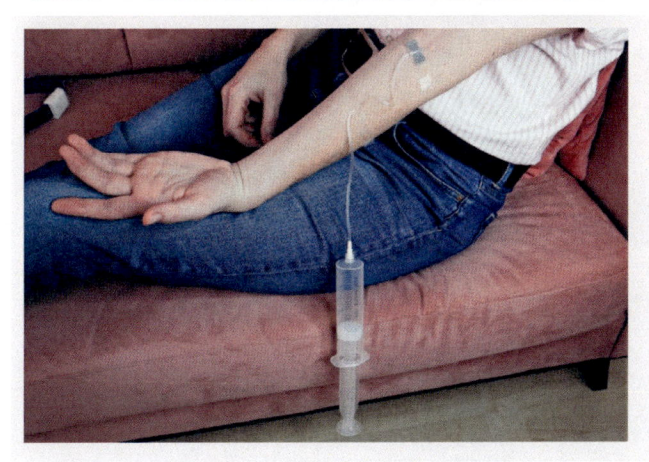

Explanation of step 10.49.
The second piece of tape secures the inserted needle: In case you accidentally drop the syringe the needle will stay in place inside the vein.

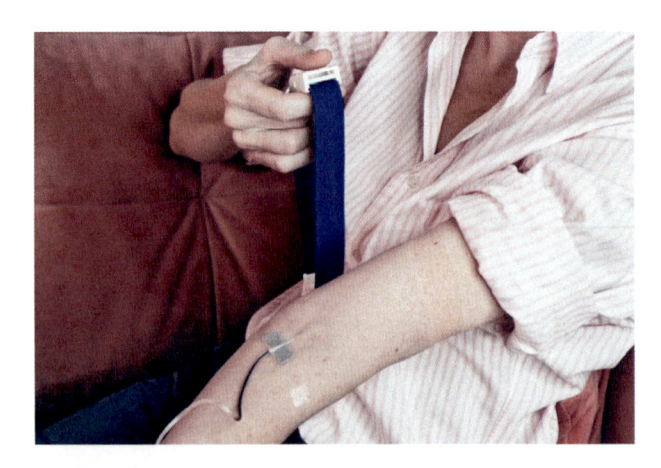

Step 10.50.

Remove the tourniquet. VERY IMPORTANT. DO NOT FORGET!!!

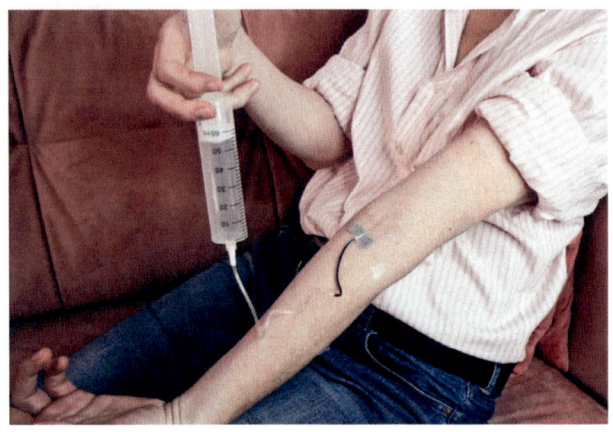

Step 10.51.

Grab the syringe with your other hand and flip it upside down.

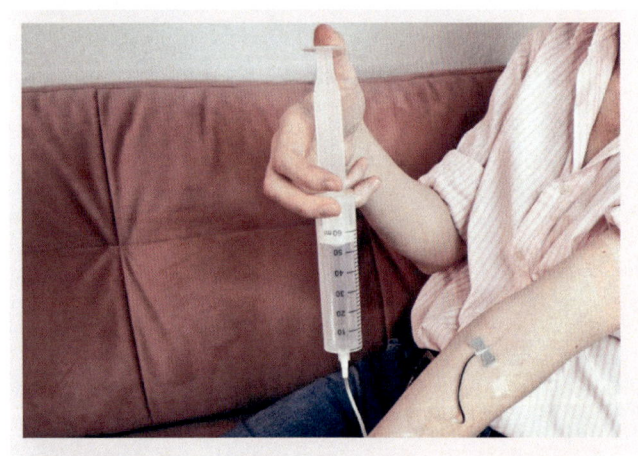

Explanation of step 10.51.

Keep the syringe flipped upside down for the duration of the injection. If, in spite of all the precautions, air got inside the syringe, it will now collect at the top, since ozone is heavier than air.

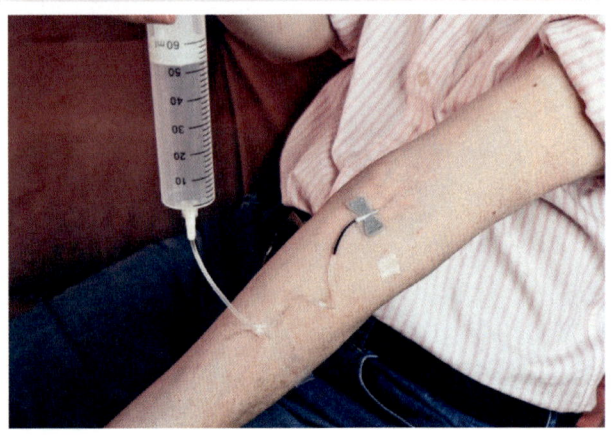

Step 10.52.

Keep pushing the plunger of the syringe until the blood is out of the line. You want to get the blood out of the butterfly line within 30 seconds. If you wait too long it will coagulate and block the line.

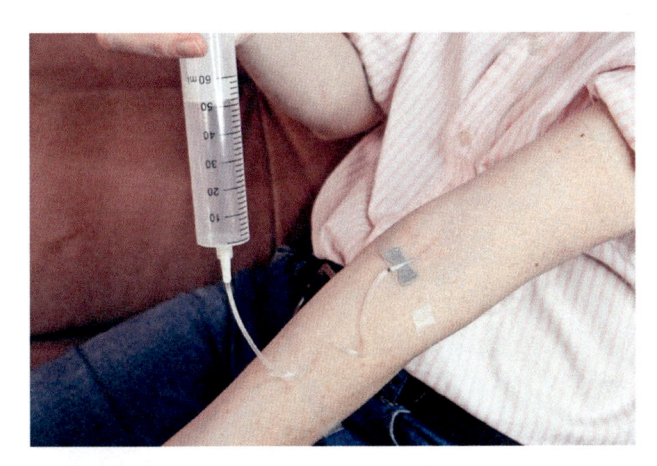

Step 10.53.
The moment the blood is out of the line, stop pushing the plunger and start counting to 20 seconds.

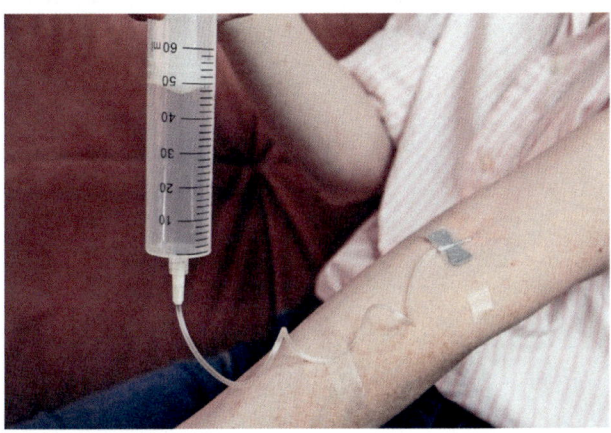

Step 10.54.
After 20 seconds push another 1 cc.

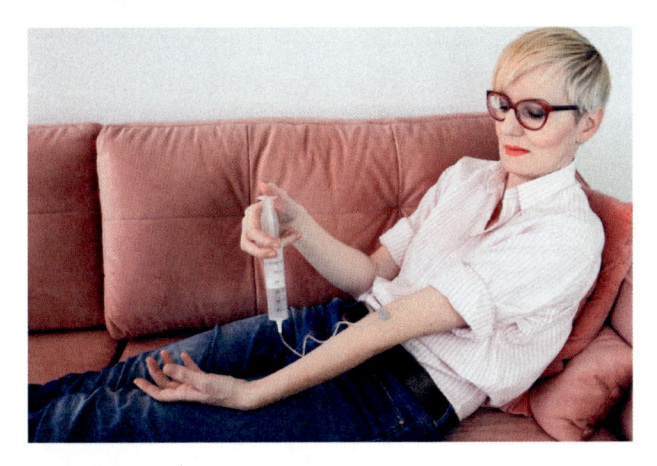

Step 10.55.
Keep repeating it at that tempo while keeping the syringe upside down the whole time. The whole injection can take between 10 and 25 minutes.

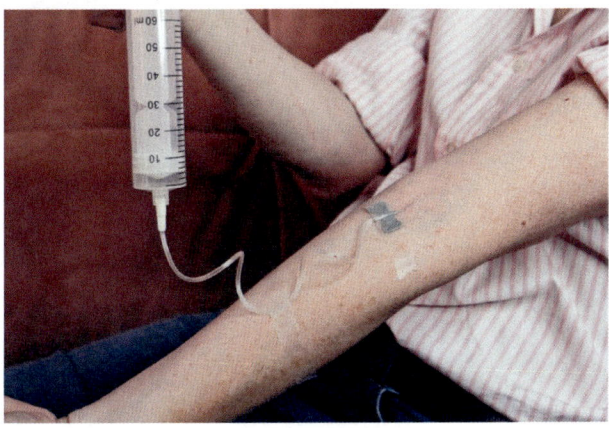

Step 10.56.
Repeat step 10.55. Until there are only 5 cc left in the syringe.

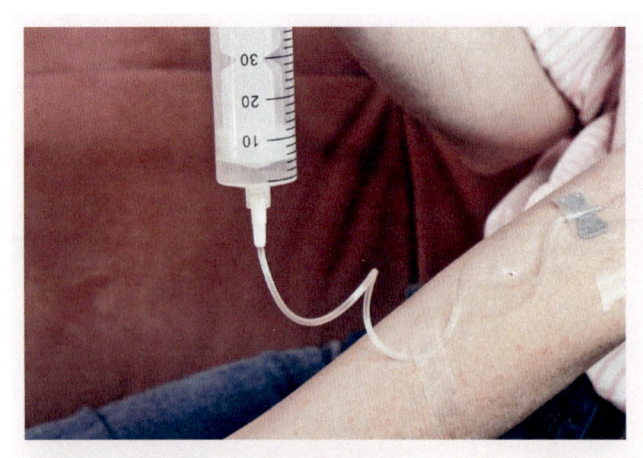

Explanation of step 10.56.
Leave 5 cc of gas inside the syringe when you are done. Those are the hypothetical 5 cc of air which may have gotten inside the syringe and which may have collected close to the plunger if you have kept the syringe vertical the whole time as directed above.

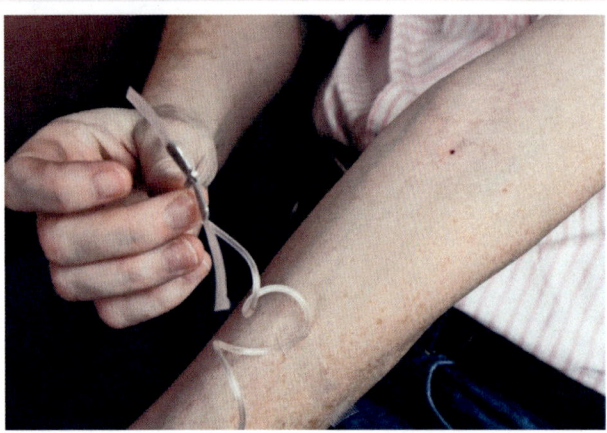

Step 10.57.
When you're done, untape the butterflies, remove the needle and the syringe.

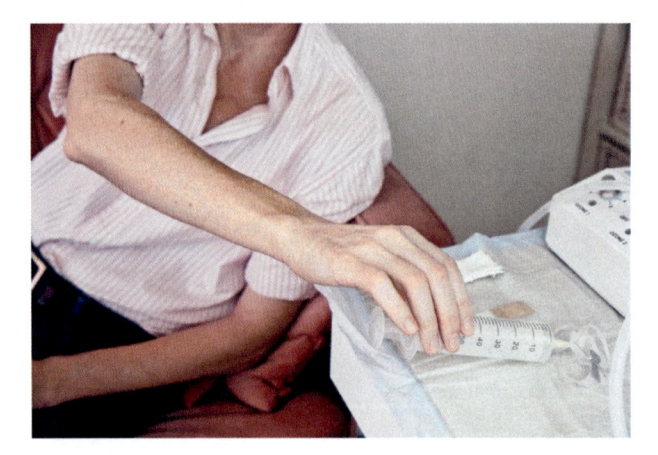

Step 10.58.
Put the syringe with the needle aside. You will take care of it later.

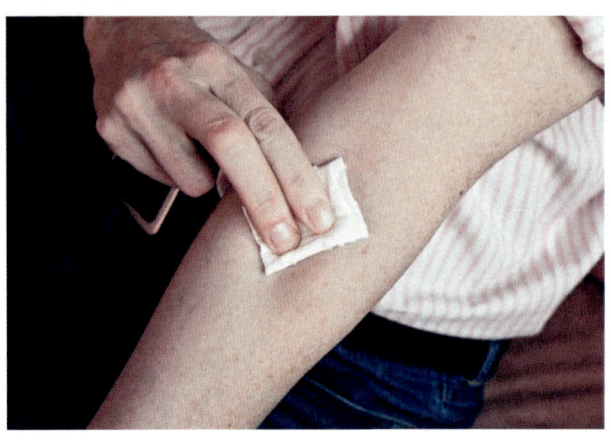

Step 10.59.
Take a cotton pad and press it on the puncture wound.

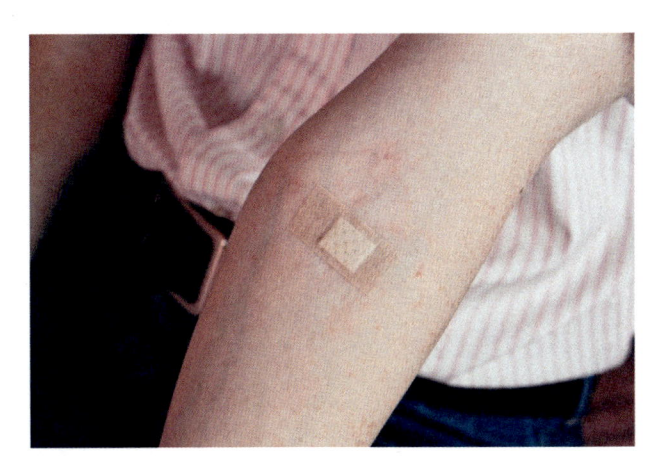

Step 10.60.
Place a bandaid on it.

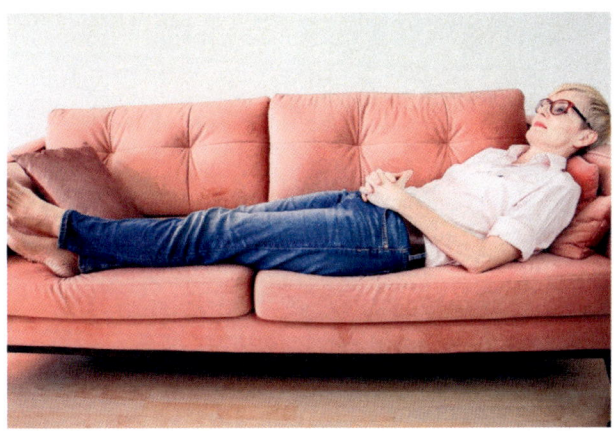

Step 10.61.
Remain reclined and immobile for at least 30 minutes. Do not laugh, do not talk, do not move your limbs. Play with your smartphone, read a book, watch TV, or meditate.

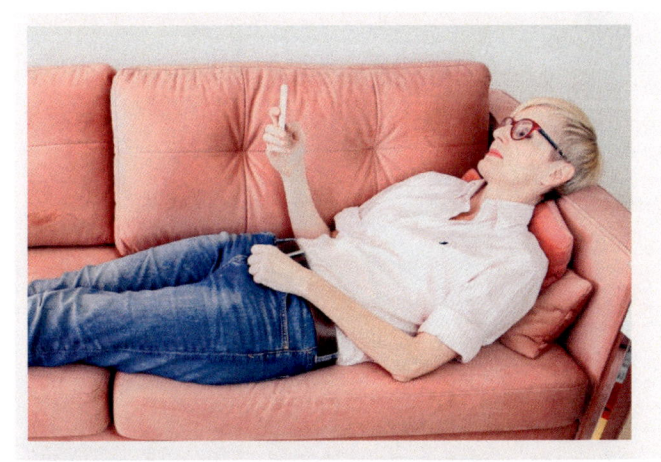

Explanation of step 10.61.
You need to allow the oxygen to be absorbed by the blood. Do not get up under any circumstances before 30 min have elapsed.

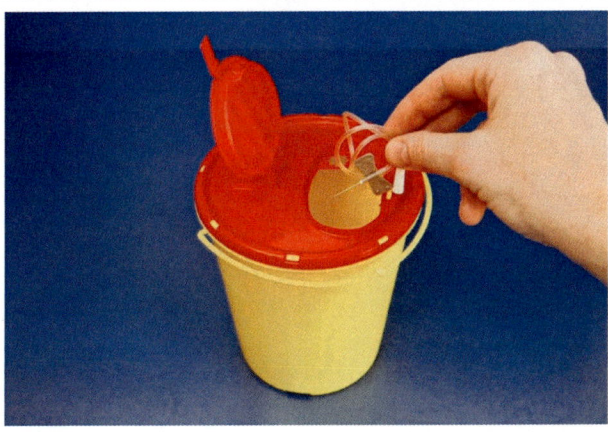

Step 10.62.
After 30 min, get up and unscrew the needle from the syringe and dispose of it in the sharps bin (or empty laundry bottle).

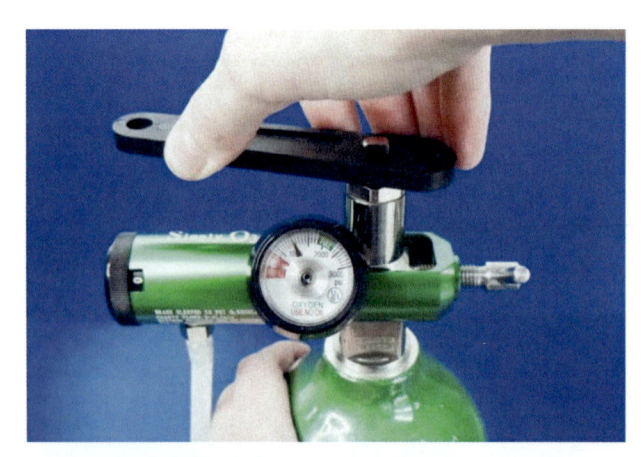

Step 10.63.
Purge the pressure from the regulator by first closing the valve on the oxygen tank.

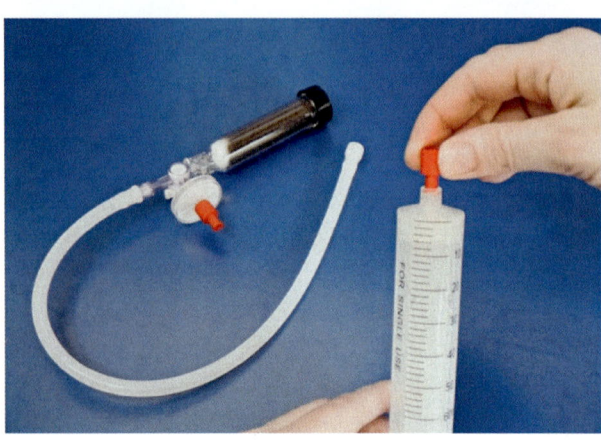

Step 10.64.
Take a sterile syringe cap and put it over the filter. Do the same with the syringe.

Chapter 10 questions

1. Describe the 4 principles upon which the "DIV for the Superparanoid" method is based.

2. After having filled the syringe and after having closed the syringe port on the filling station, what is the immediate next step? (Only one correct answer)

    a) Unscrew syringe.
    b) Turn off everything: the ozone generator and the regulator.
    c) Keep syringe vertical.

3. You finished the injection and you pulled the needle out of your arm, what do you do next? (Only one correct answer)

    a) I remain in a horizontal, immoble, stretched out position for at least 30 minutes.
    b) I dispose of the needle.
    c) I close the tank and purge the pressure from the regulator.

4. Why is it important to hold the syringe port of the syringe filling station pointing up after unscrewing the syringe? (step 10.16.)?

5. Why is it important to hold the syringe filling station up and let the syringe be vertical, before unscrewing it? (steps 10.27., 10.28.)

6. You have successfully punctured the vein and you have taped down the butterflies and the line of the butterfly needle, what is the next step? (only one correct answer).
    a) Press the plunger of the syringe until there is no more visible blood in the line.
    b) Remove the tourniquet.
    c) Flip the syringe upside down.

7. Why is it important to not let the needle dangle after having purged the line of the butterfly needle?

Sources
[1] Kreutzer, Franz J.: "Intravenöse Sauerstofftherapie (IOT)", 2014

11. How to inject more than 60 cc

As long as no chest tightness occurs, more than 60 ml of oxygen/ozone gas mix can be injected in one session. To achieve this, several syringes are used. They are filled in advance and then switched out at the end of each injection. Typically, not more than 120 ml, or two syringe fills are used, although I've heard of a case where 400 ml were injected during one treatment. **As long as there is no chest tightness, more than 60 cc of gas can be infused.**

If more than 60 cc are injected, it's recommended to use a 25g butterfly instead of 27g to prevent clogging of the needle during the swap. You will also need a tall glass or cup.

Step-by-step procedure

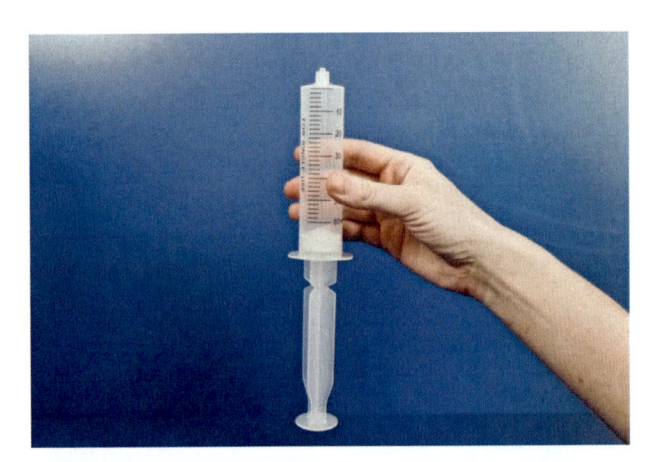

Step 11.1.
Fill a syringe with ozone following steps 10.1. to 10.29. Choose a slightly higher ozone concentration (by ca. 20%) to account for the time delay.

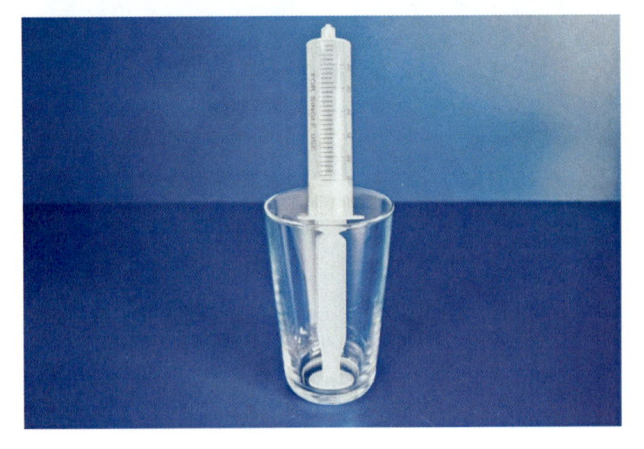

Step 11.2.
Place the syringe inside a glass - upright. Place it close to where you will be lying to make it easy to grab the syringe without having to get up. Put an extra cap on the syringe, if you want.

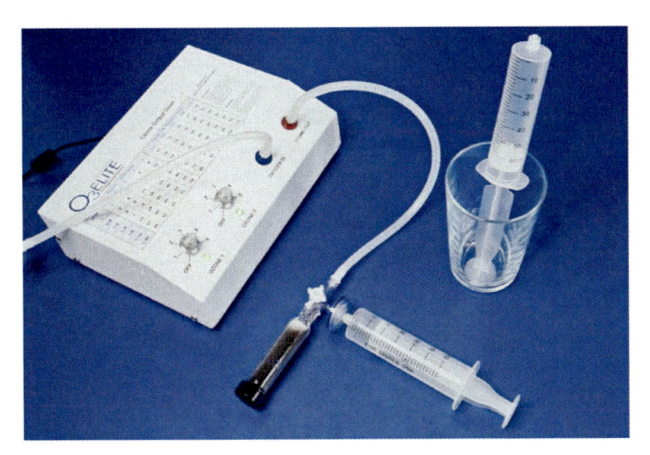

Step 11.3.
Fill the second syringe according to steps 10.1. to 10.29. This is the one you will use first, so fill it with the normal ozone concentration.

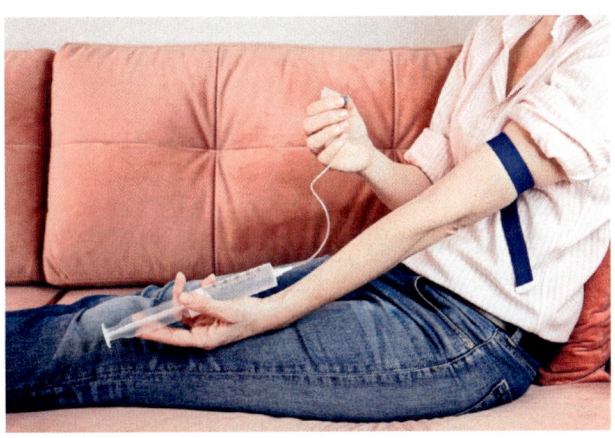

Step 11.4.
Perform the injection according to steps 10.30. to 10.55.

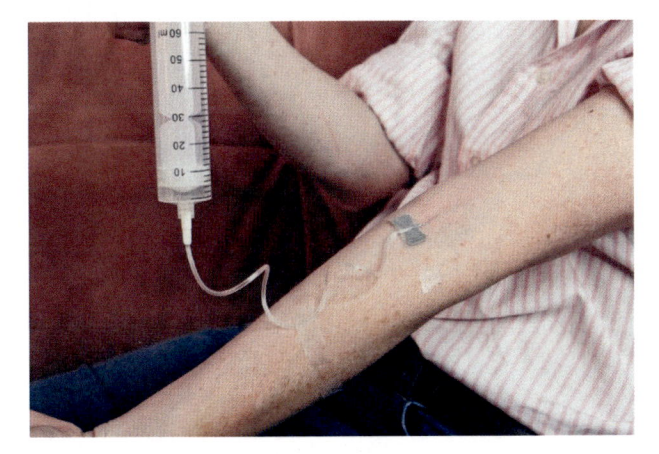

Step 11.5.
Once you arrive at step 10.55. with only 5 cc left, it's time to switch the syringes.

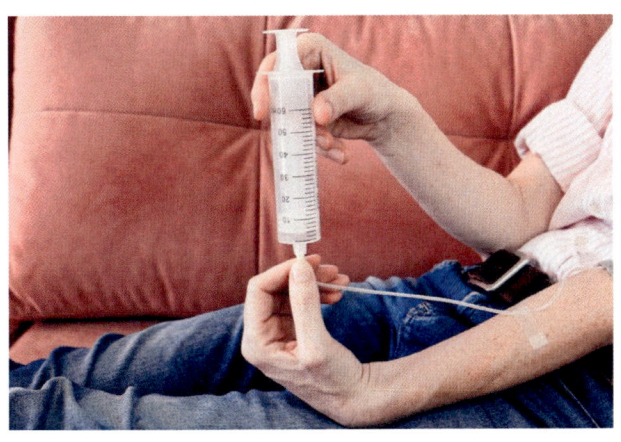

Step 11.6.
Grab the end of the butterfly line with the syringe still attached to it and hold it upright.

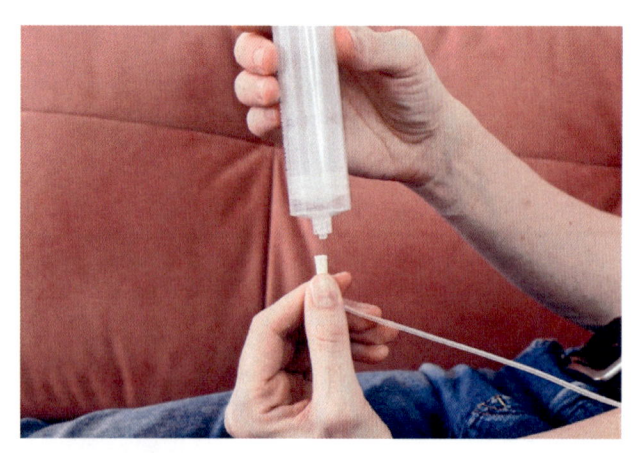

Step 11.7.
Unscrew the syringe. Keep the open end of the butterfly line up all the time to make sure no ozone pours out.

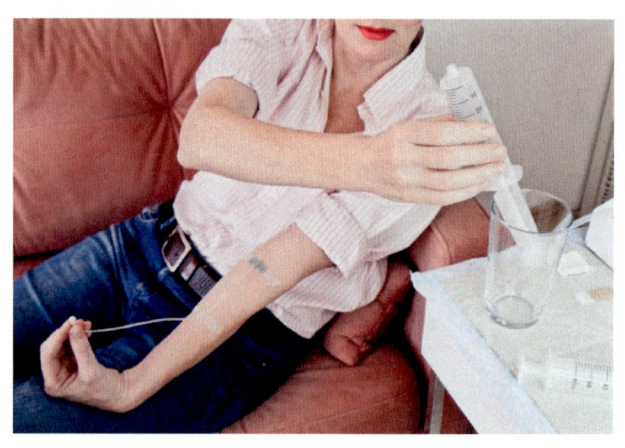

Step 11.8.
Grab the second syringe. Keep holding the butterfly line up.

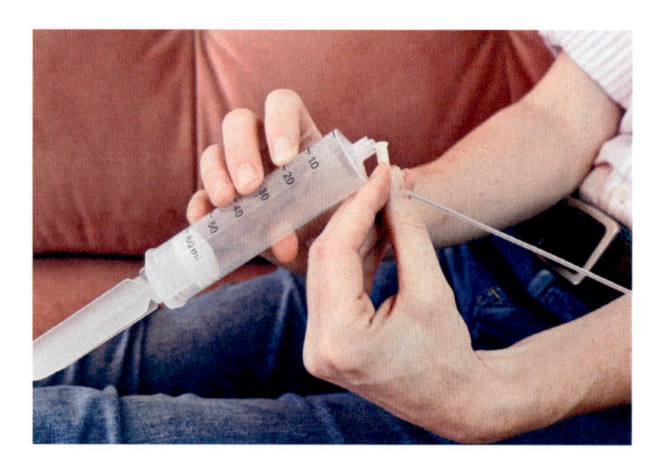

Step 11.9.
Move the new syringe as close as possible to the butterfly line.

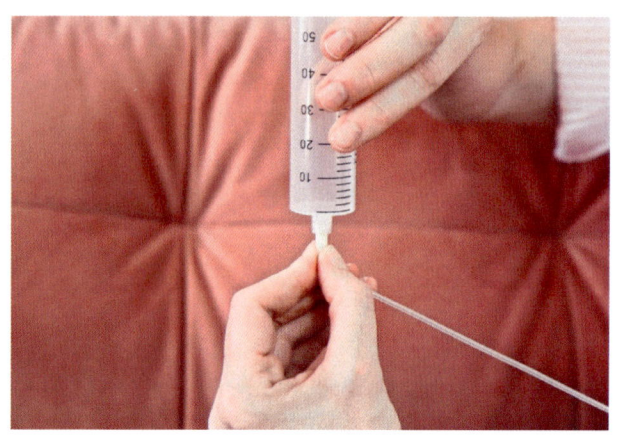

Step 11.10.
With one quick movement flip the syringe ...

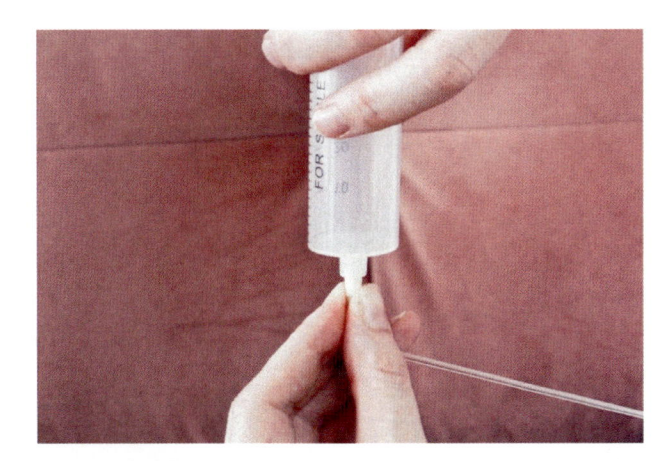

Step 11.11.
… and screw onto the butterfly line.

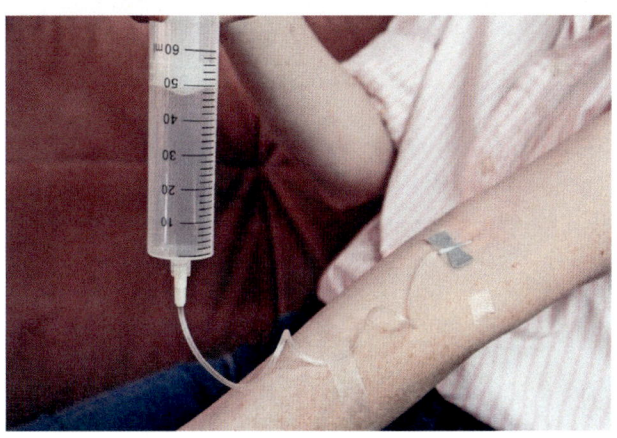

Step 11.12.
Proceed as you would before by pushing 1 cc every 20 seconds. Finish the injection according to steps 10.53. to 10.65.

Chapter 11 questions

1. Describe the process of attaching a second syringe, once you are done injecting the content of the first one.
2. Why should you fill the second syringe with a slightly higher ozone concentration?
3. In which position should the second syringe be placed before it's used?

12. How to treat varicose veins with DIV injections

Varicose veins can be treated very successfully with DIV ozone injections. Both the blue discoloration as well as the bulging of the vein can be completely eliminated, often with just one injection. To accomplish this, a relatively high ozone concentration of 50 to 70 mcg/ml is selected.

The injection is performed just like a DIV ozone injection with all the precautions and safety steps described in chapter 10.

Since here the lower extremities are injected instead of the upper ones, it's important to make sure that legs are stretched out and not kinked. This is crucial to keep the blood flow unimpaired. Bent legs could cause a built-up and sudden release of gas which then could cause serious complications.

After the injection you can expect a painful swelling of the vein for 3 to 4 days. The injection will trigger inflammation, or phlebitis. During this time it can become very painful to walk. After the phlebitis has resolved, the vein will have lost its discoloration and bulging.

The result can last several months to several years and can be repeated as often as needed.

Special considerations

When performing DIV ozone injections to treat varicose veins, consider the following important points:

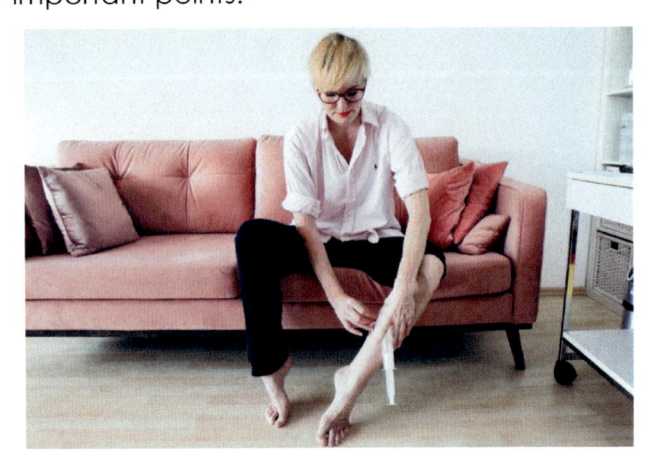

Inject while sitting or standing

You may have to inject the vein in a sitting or standing position to be able to see the vein. After the puncture, tape the needle and the line down, and then move to a reclined and stretched out position.

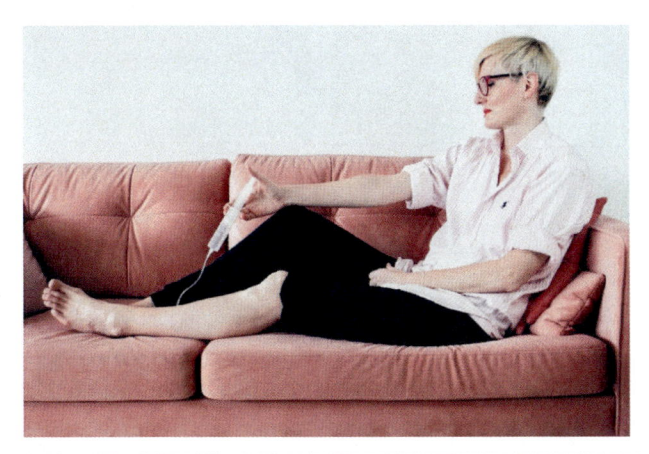

Make sure you are stretched out during the injection. Do not bend or kink your legs when pushing the gas in.

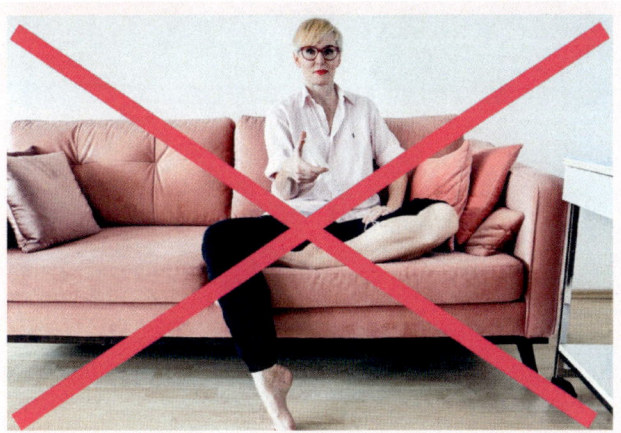

Do not keep legs kinked or bent when injecting varicose veins. Bending your leg can impair blood flow, and cause a larger gas built-up. Always keep your body stretched out when performing DIV ozone injections.

Before / After Pictures
The below pictures show before and after results when treating varicose veins with DIV ozone treatments. Although some after pictures were taken under a different lighting, one can still see significant results.

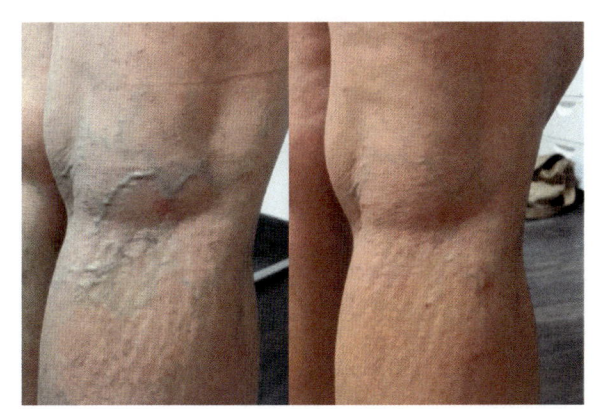

Picture on the right shows the result after 2 to 3 DIVs.   *This is the result of just one DIV ozone injection.*

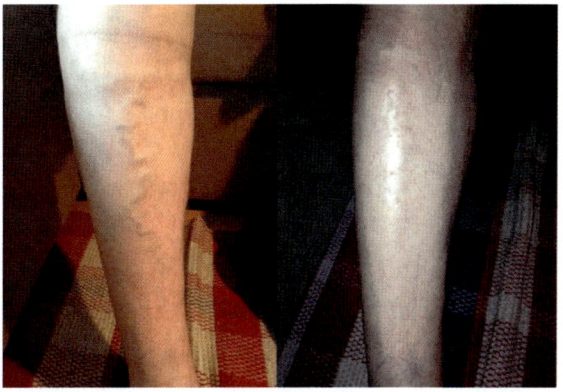

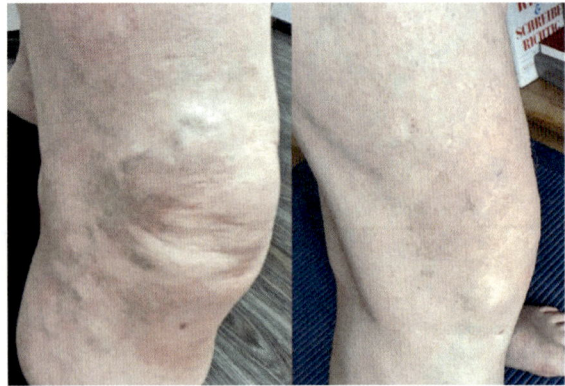

This is the result of around 2 DIV ozone injections.

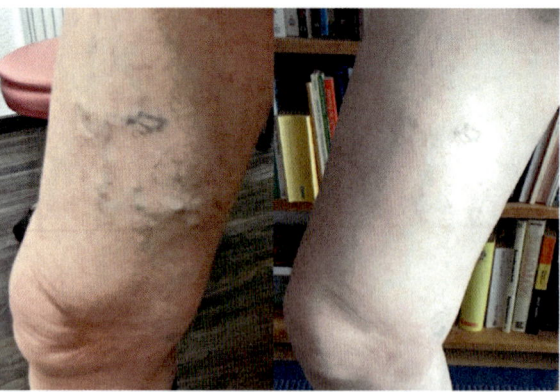

Picture on the right is the result of several DIVs.

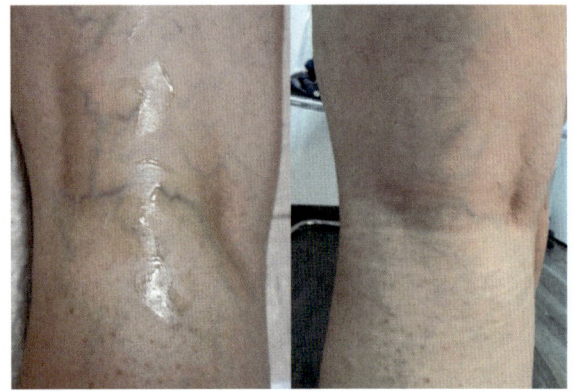

Left is the before picture with the anesthetic cream applied. Picture on the right displays a significant improvement.

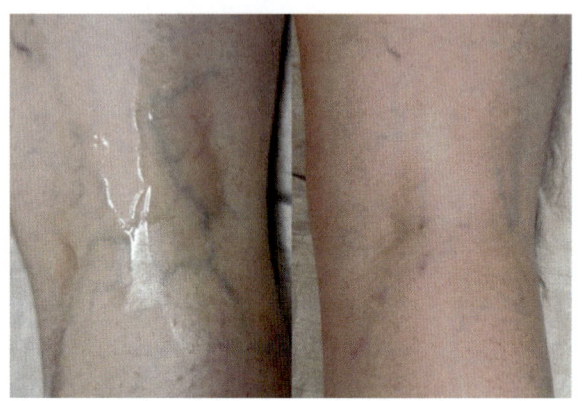

Picture on the right shows the result immediately after the injection.

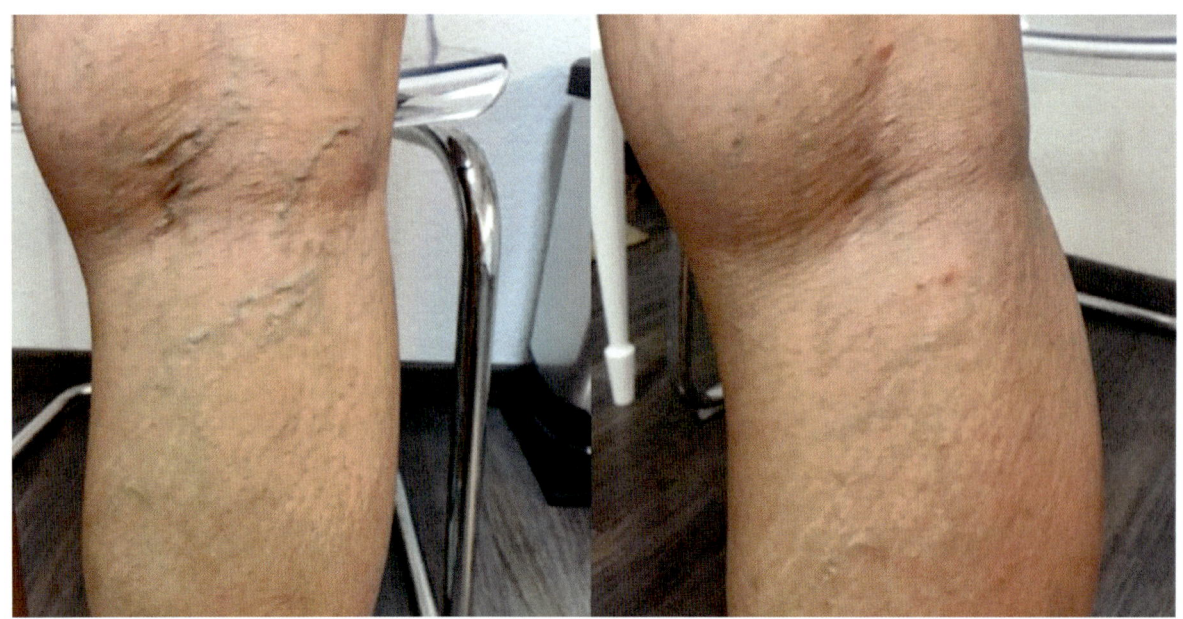

Same leg as the first picture, but a different angle. One can see the complete disappearance of the most pronounced veins.

Chapter 12 questions

1. What is the recommended ozone concentration to treat varicose veins?
2. How should your body be positioned when you inject varicose veins on your legs?
3. What is to be expected right after the injections?

13. How to perform DIV with a glass syringe

Using a glass syringe is not part of the "DIV for the Superparanoid" method. Handling a glass syringe increases the risk of air contamination considerably. Especially for beginners, a glass syringe is not recommended. But even advanced DIV administrators can have trouble with it.

For those who are willing to take the risk, in this chapter I show what I believe is one of the safest methods for handling a glass syringe during DIV ozone injections.

You will need the following two additional accessories:

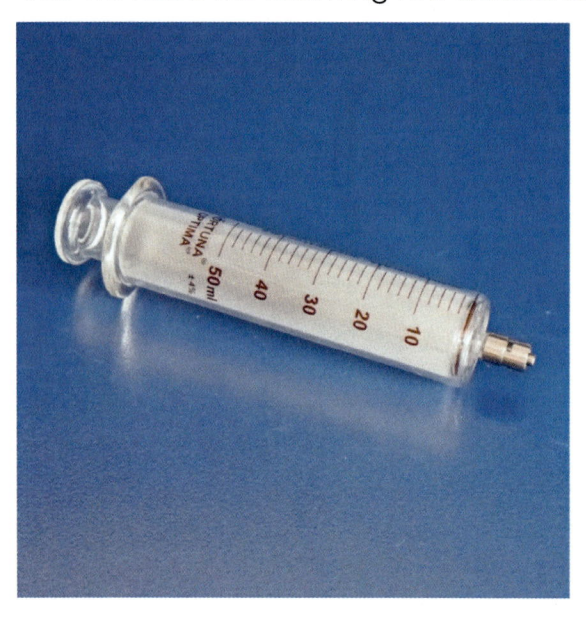

A 50 ml glass syringe with a luer lock attachment.

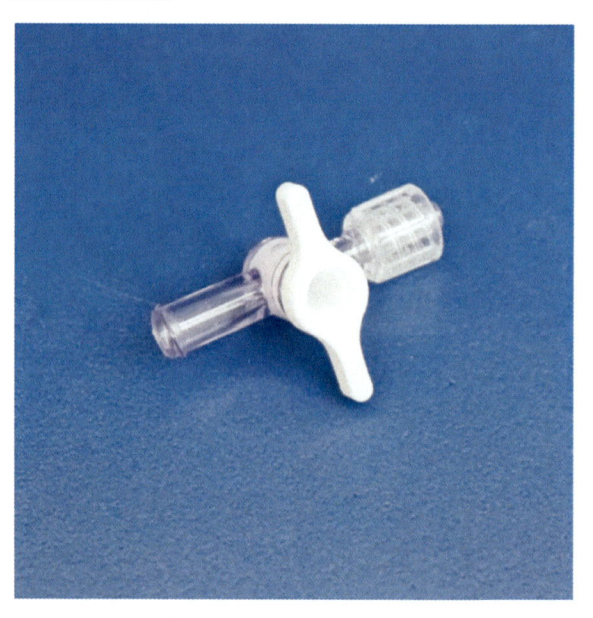

This is an ON / OFF valve, since it has two settings: on or off. It can block or open the gas flow.

When working with a glass syringe, two different valves are used: a three-way-valve (which is part of the syringe filling station) and the ON/OFF valve. So, the process involves the logical coordination of the settings of the two different valves.

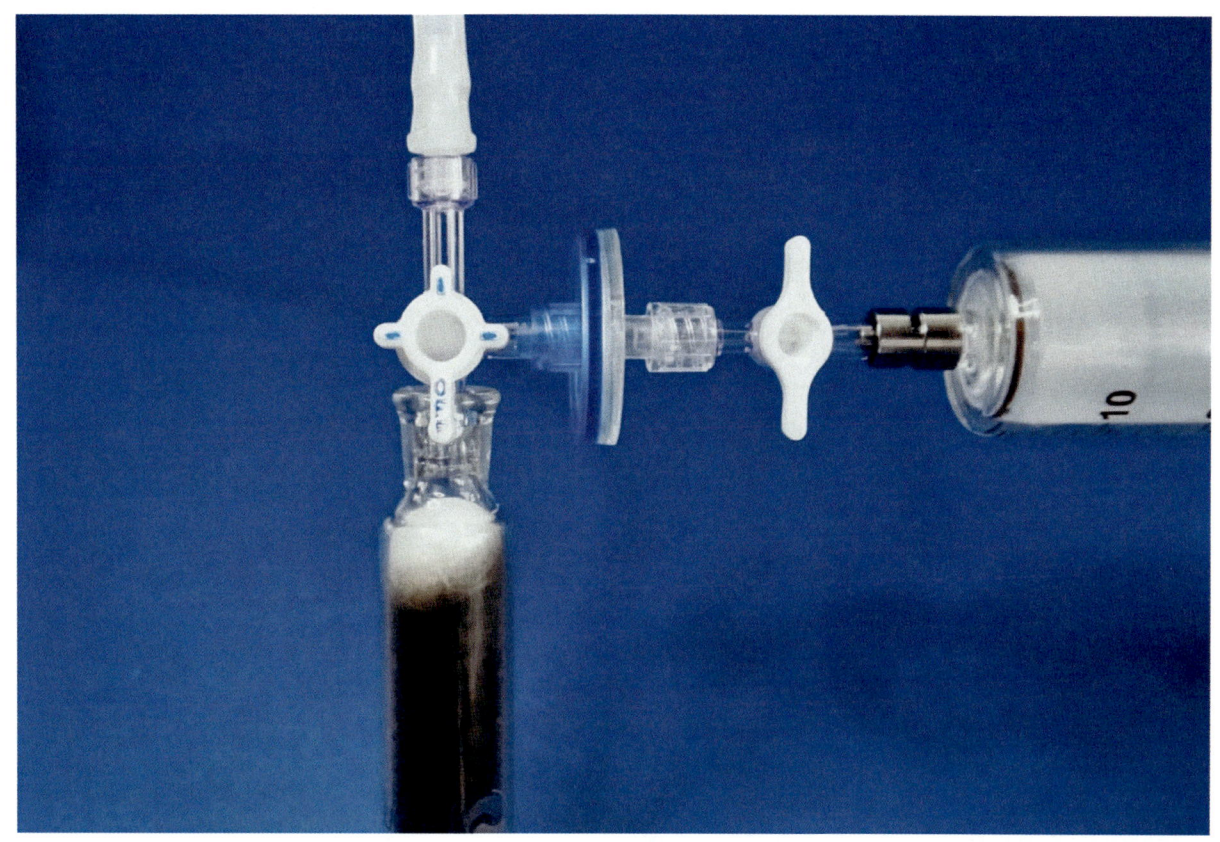

At the heart of the glass syringe filling system are two different valves: a three way and a two-way (ON/OFF) valve with a filter in between.

If at a certain point one of the valves is turned to the wrong position, a blockage of the gas flow will occur and pressure will build up. This will result in a sudden disconnect of one of the silicone tubings.

To prevent this, it's of utmost importance to follow the exact settings of the two valves as laid out in the steps below.

Step-by-step procedure
Before starting the procedure, read chapters 3 and 4, and prepare everything according to chapters 6, 7, and 8.

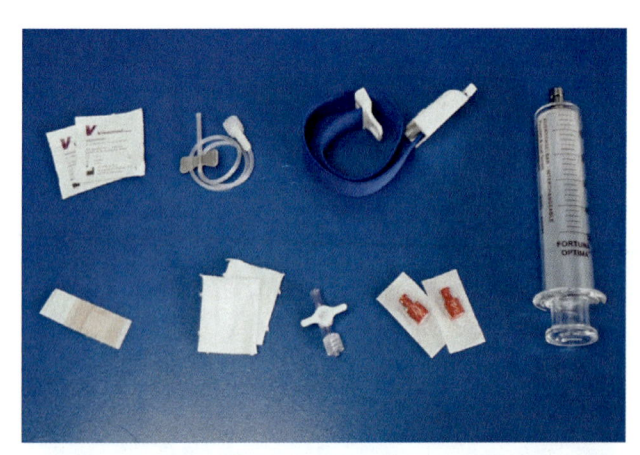

Step 13.1.
Prepare all the supplies: alcohol wipes, butterfly needle, tourniquet, band-aid, cotton pads, ON/OFF valve, syringe caps, glass syringe.

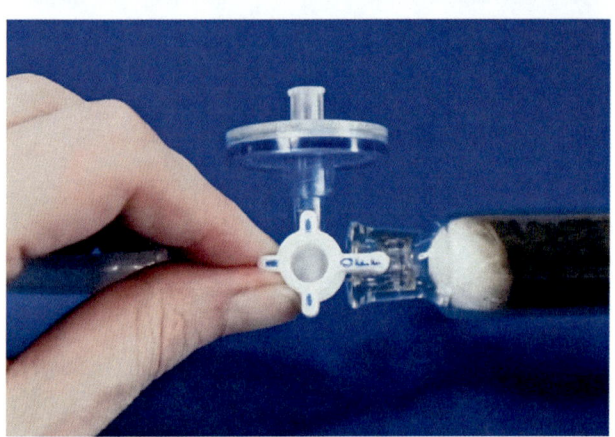

Step 13.2.
Proceed according to steps 10.3. to 10.10.

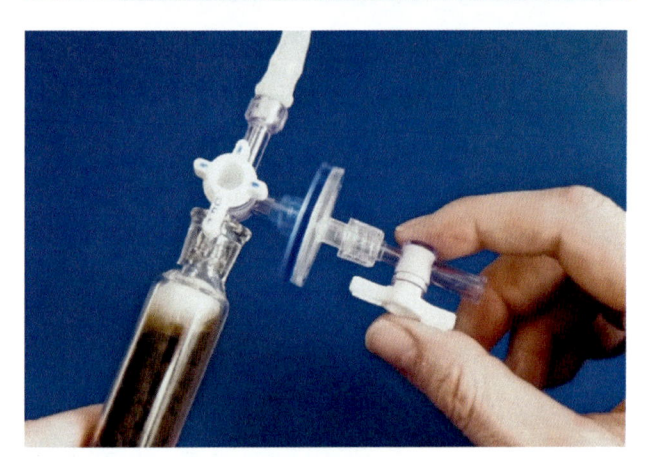

Step 13.3.
Attach the ON/OFF valve to the filter of the syringe filling station. Make sure the valve is open, or ON.

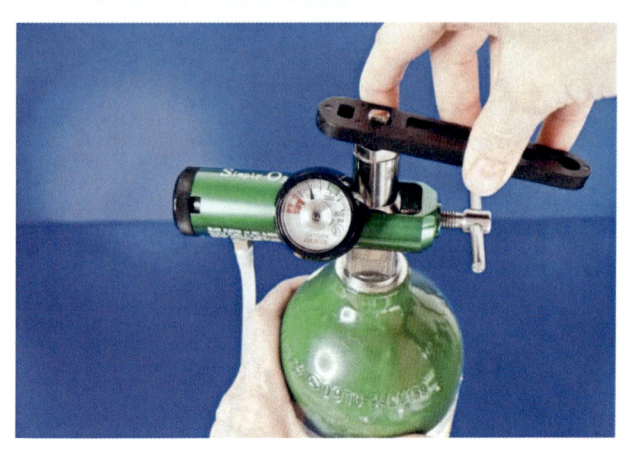

Step 13.4.
Open the valve on the tank. Half a turn is enough. Watch the gauge jump up.

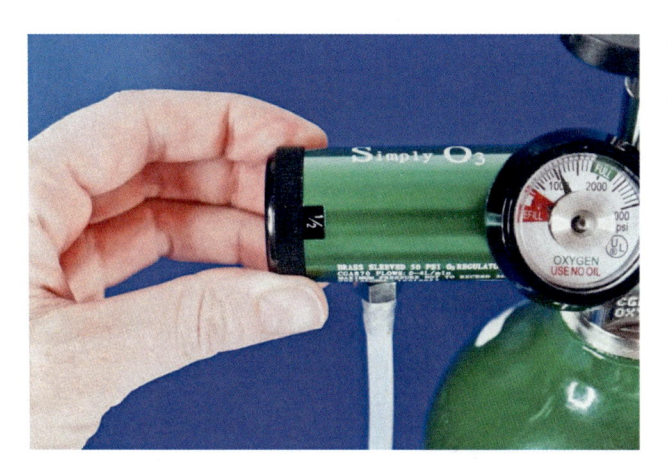

Step 13.5.
Open the regulator to 1/2 LPM.

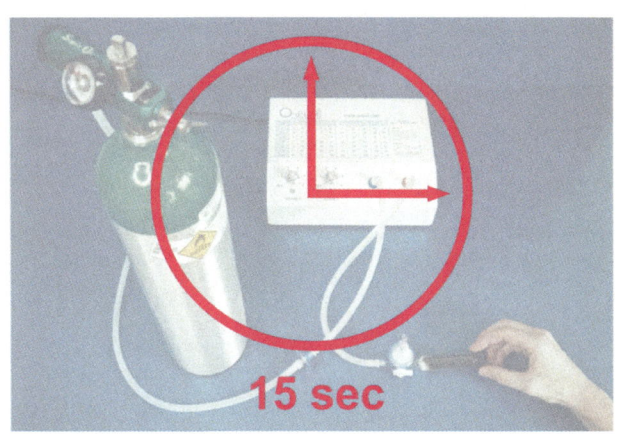

Step 13.6.
Count 15 seconds. This will flush all the lines with pure oxygen. Hold the filling station pointing up while you do so.

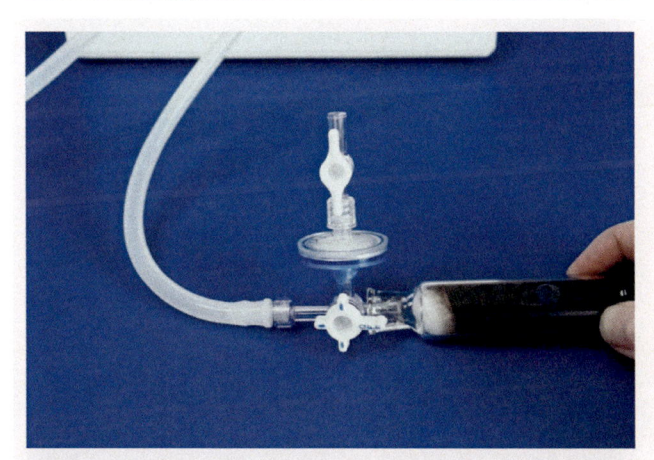

Explanation of step 13.6.
Make sure that during the flushing the syringe port points up, otherwise the oxygen could flow out and air could enter.

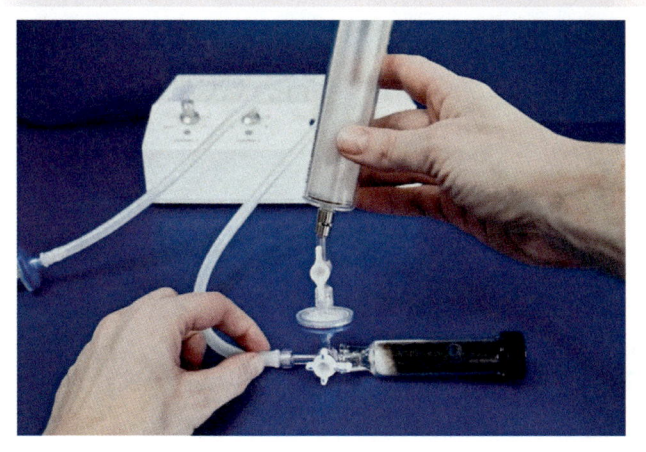

Step 13.7.
Screw the glass syringe on to flush it with pure oxygen.

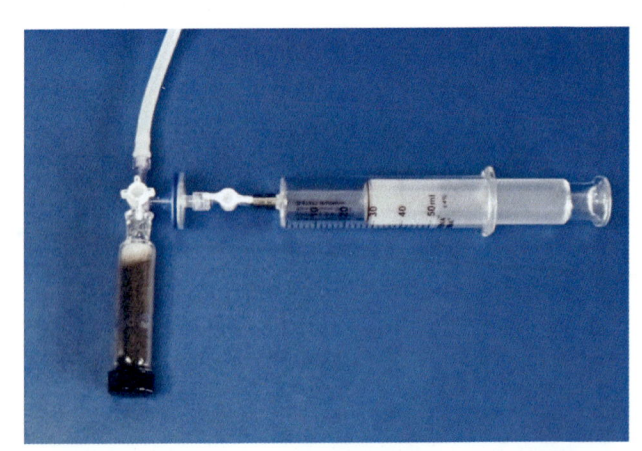

Step 13.8.
Fill the syringe with oxygen. Watch out, it will go quickly. You can let go of the filling station during this step.

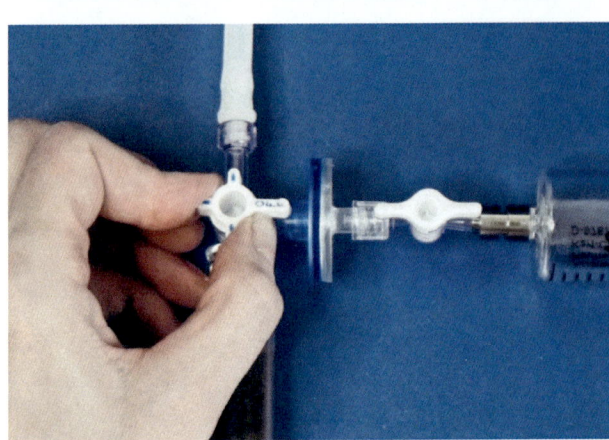

Step 13.9.
When the syringe is full, turn the OFF lever towards the syringe port to close it. The ON/OFF valve remains open.

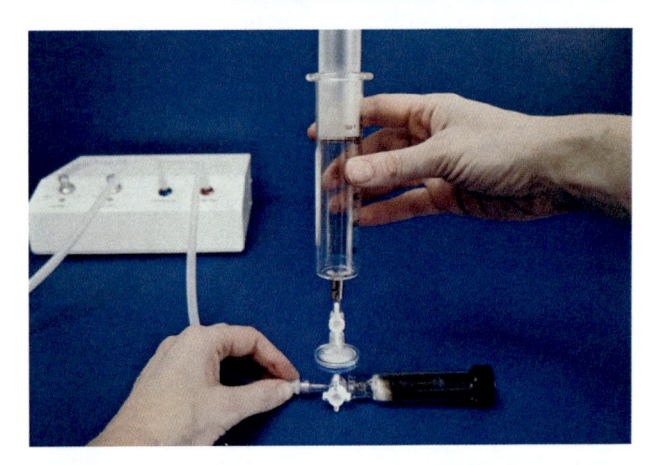

Step 13.10.
Flip the syringe filling station so that the syringe is vertical and upside down.

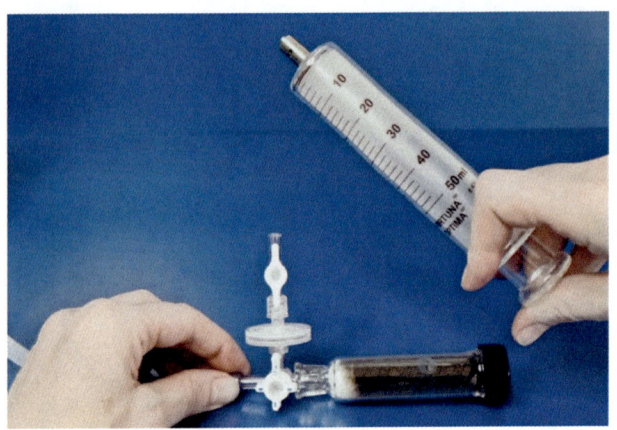

Step 13.11.
Unscrew and empty the syringe all the while keeping the filling station pointing up.

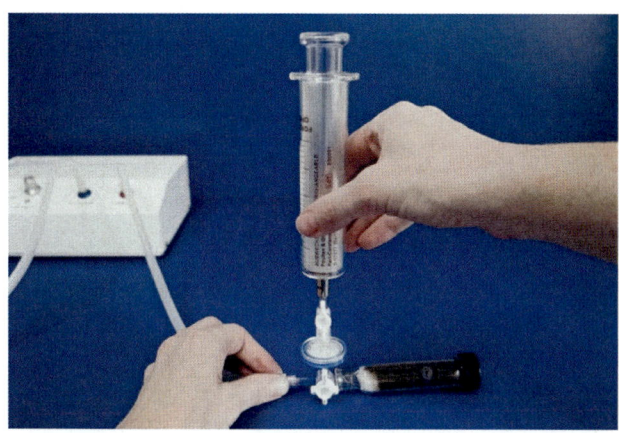

Step 13.12.
Screw the syringe back onto the filling station while holding the station so that the filter points up.

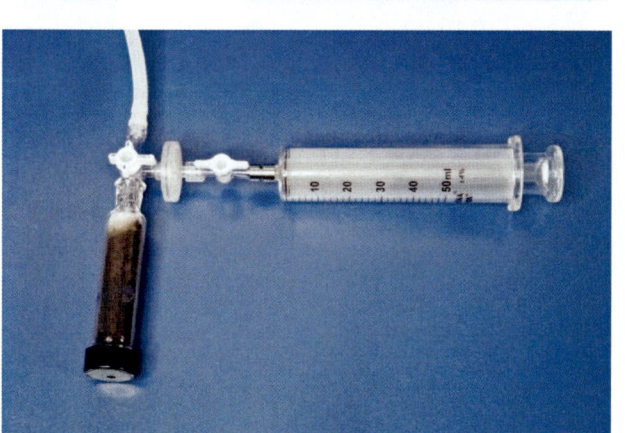

Step 13.13.
You can now let go of the filling station again.

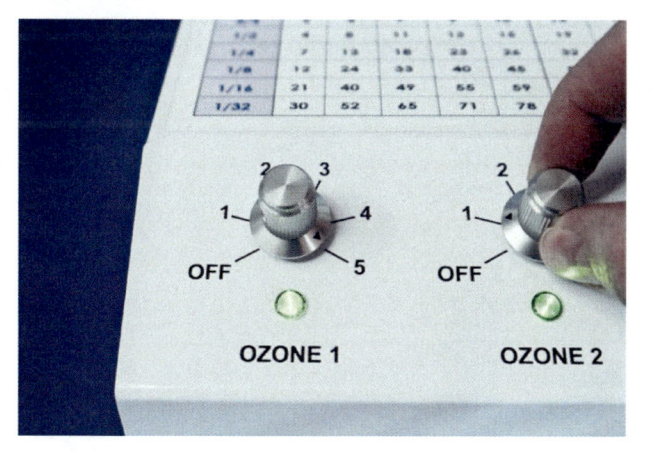

Step 13.14.
Select your ozone concentration on the ozone generator.

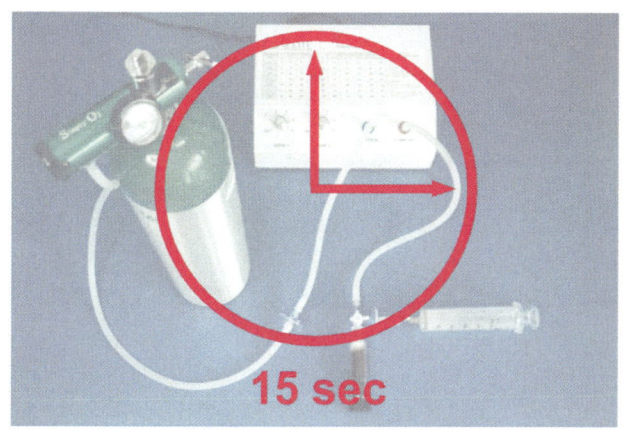

Step 13.15.
Let the ozone run for 15 sec to allow the machine to warm up and for the ozone gas to flush the lines.

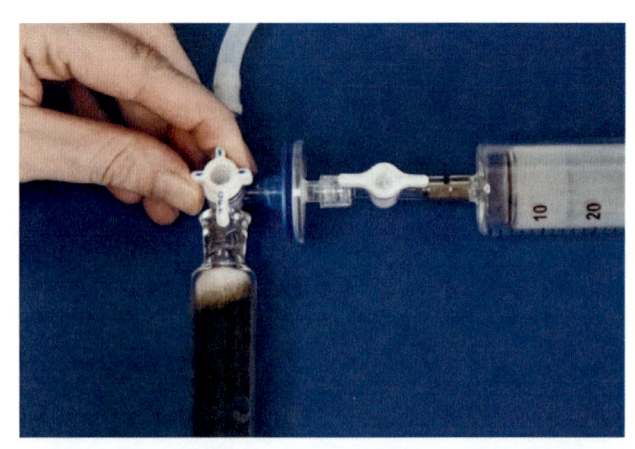

Step 13.16.
Open the valve on the syringe filling station by turning the OFF lever towards the destructor.

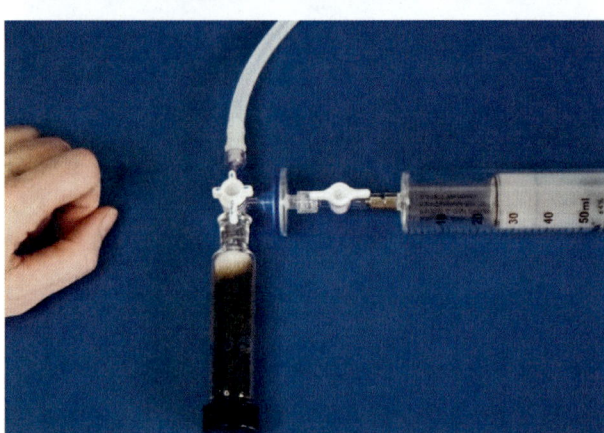

Step 13.17.
Fill the syringe. It will go fast, so keep your hand close. Fill it to the last mark, in this case 50 ml. Do not go beyond it.

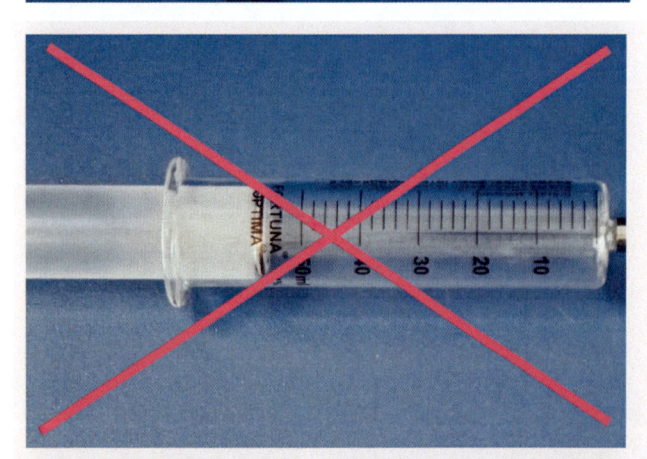

Explanation of step 13.17.
Glass syringes tend to not be airtight anymore beyond the last marking.

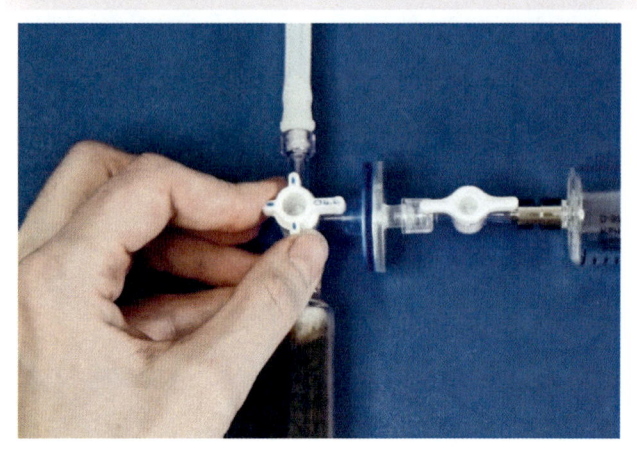

Step 13.18.
When the syringe is full, close the syringe port by turning the OFF lever towards the syringe.

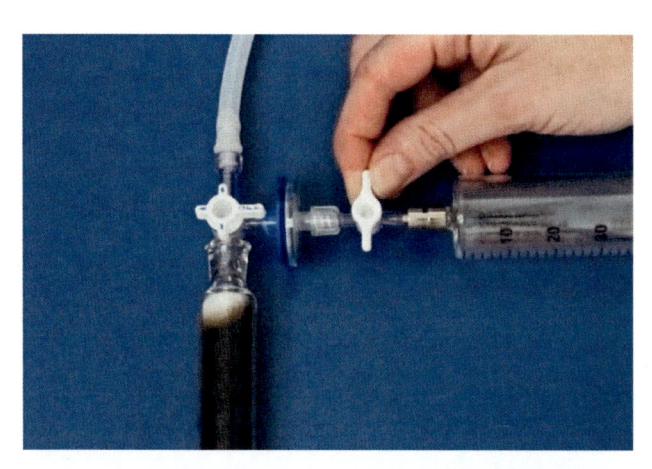

Step 13.19.
Close the ON/OFF valve.

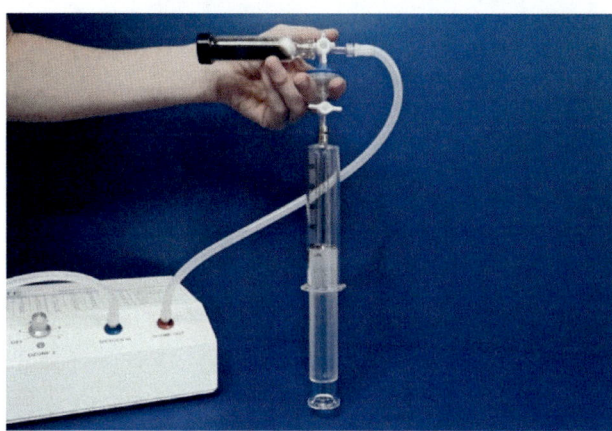

Step 13.20.
Lift the syringe filling station so that the syringe is in a vertical position.

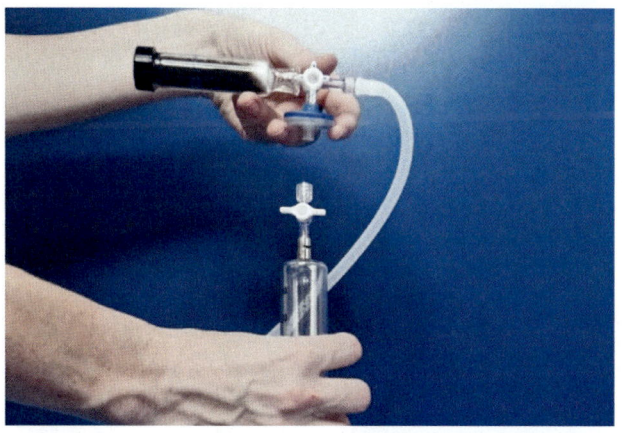

Step 13.21.
Unscrew the ON/OFF valve with the syringe attached to it, while keeping the filling station vertically the whole time.

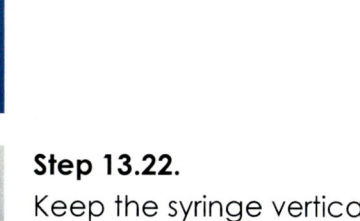

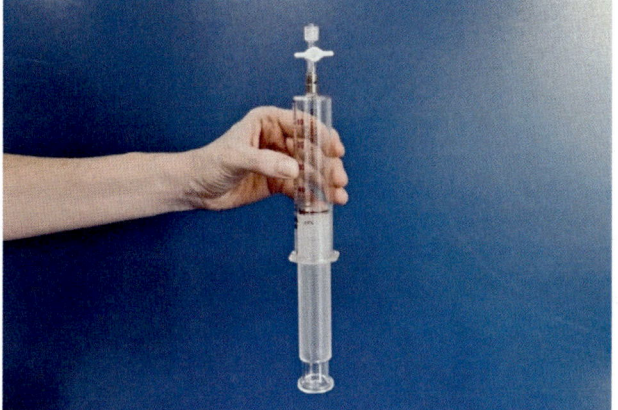

Step 13.22.
Keep the syringe vertical at all times. Do not lay it down, and do not flip it.

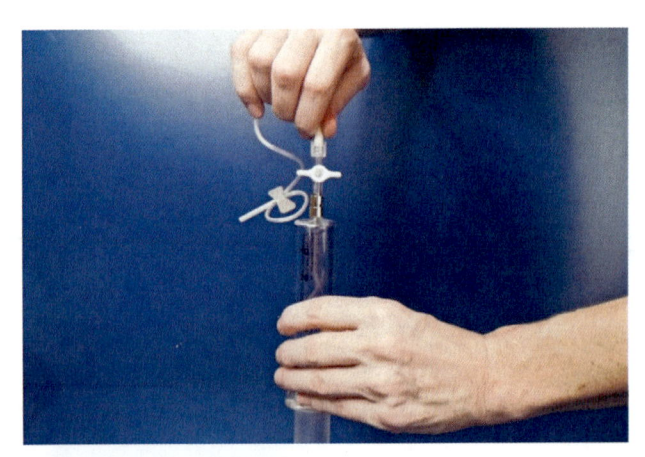

Step 13.23.
Screw the butterfly needle onto the ON/OFF valve.

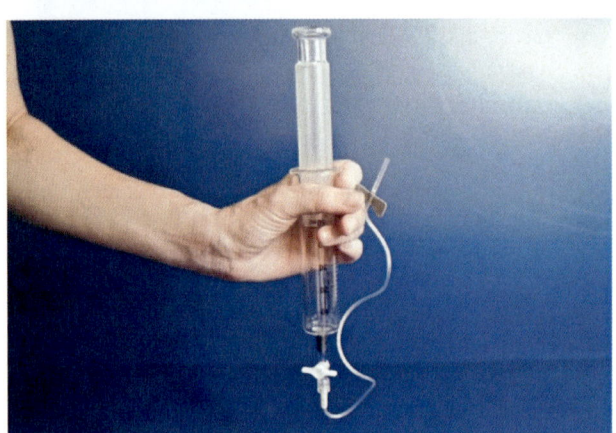

Step 13.24.
Now, flip the syringe upside down. Keep the wings of the butterfly needle between thumb and index finger.

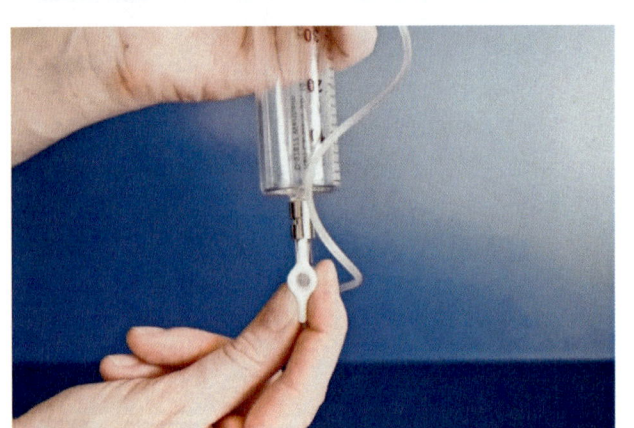

Step 13.25.
Open the ON/OFF valve.

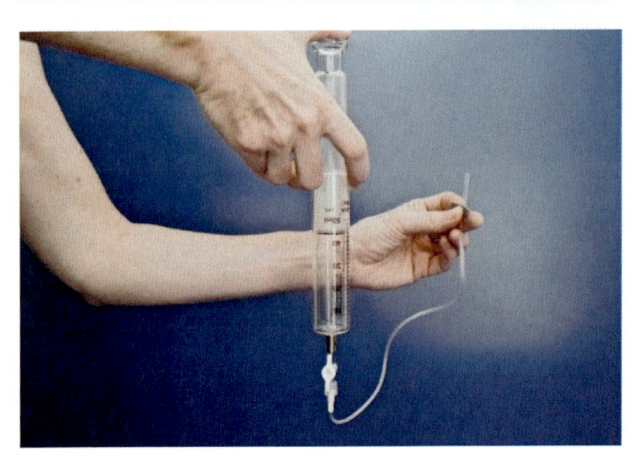

Step 13.26.
Press down on the plunger to press out around 5 ml. This will flush the line of the butterfly needle with pure ozone/oxygen mix.

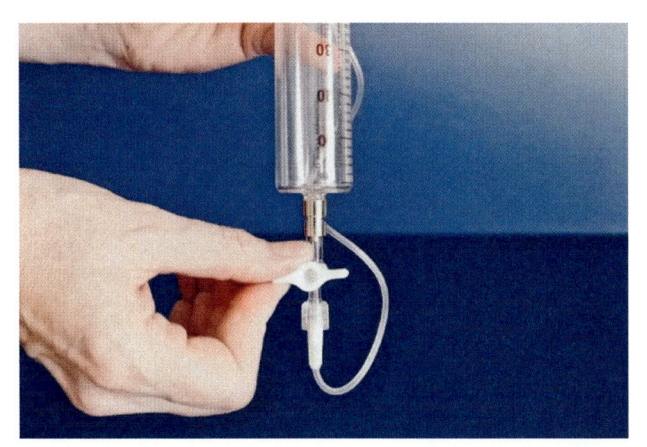

Step 13.27.
Close the ON/OFF valve.

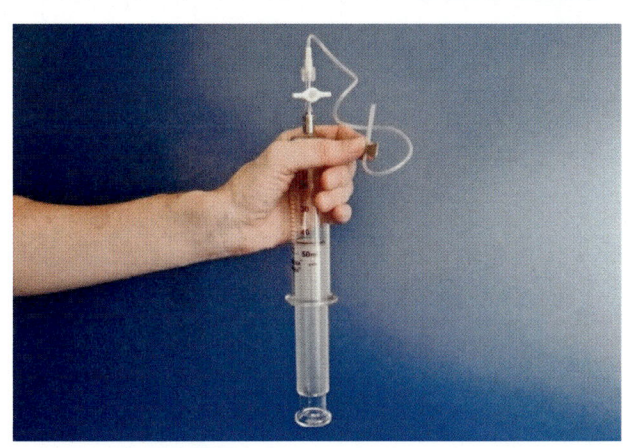

Step 13.28.
Flip the syringe upright again. Hold the butterfly needle level with the top of the syringe. Do not let the butterfly needle dangle.

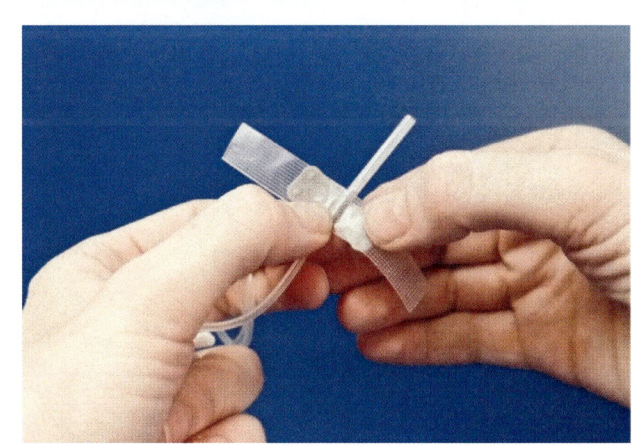

Step 13.29.
Take a piece of tape and tape it over the wings on the side with the ridge.

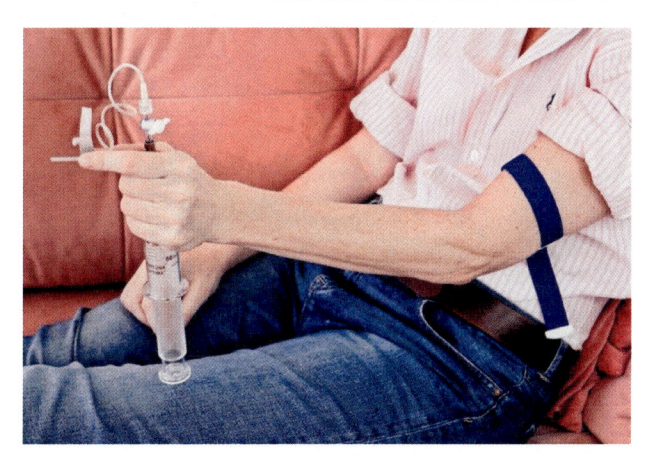

Step 13.30.
Move to where you will perform the injection. Keep holding the syringe upright.

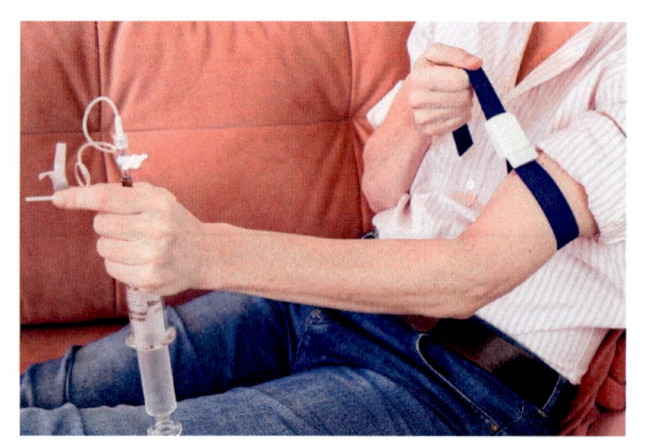

Step 13.31.
Tighten the tourniquet.

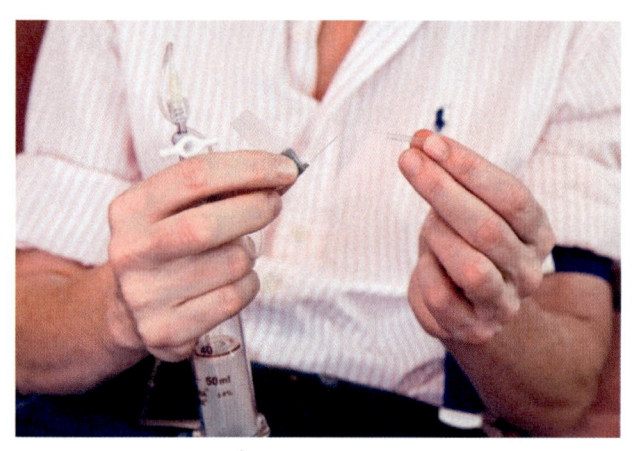

Step 13.32.
Switch the syringe into your dominant hand and remove the cap from the needle.

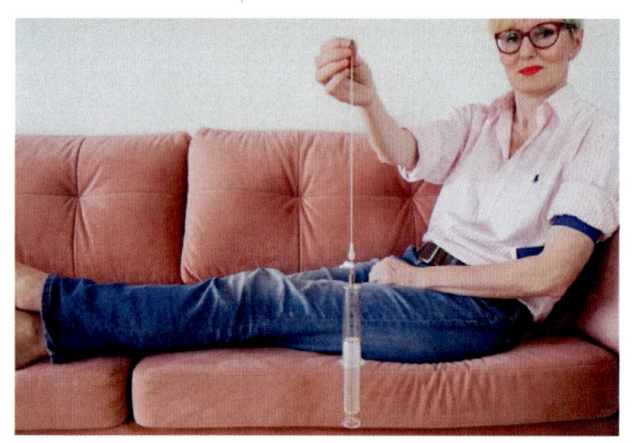

Step 13.33.
Prepare to lay the syringe into your non-dominant hand: keep holding the butterflies firmly in your dominant hand and let the syringe dangle.

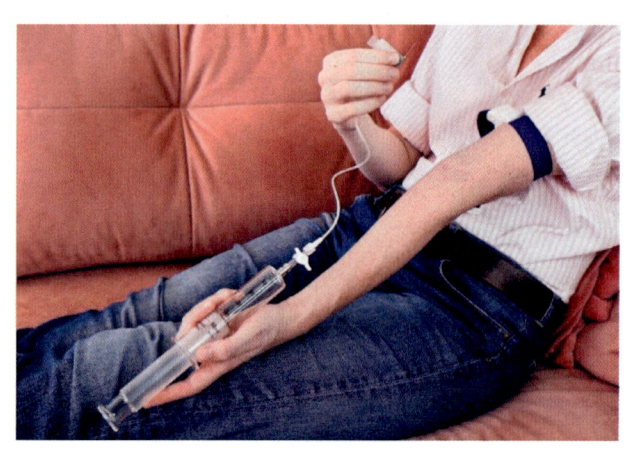

Step 13.34.
Now lay the syringe onto the palm of your non-dominant hand. Up until the injection, the needle always stays above the syringe to prevent ozone from pouring out.

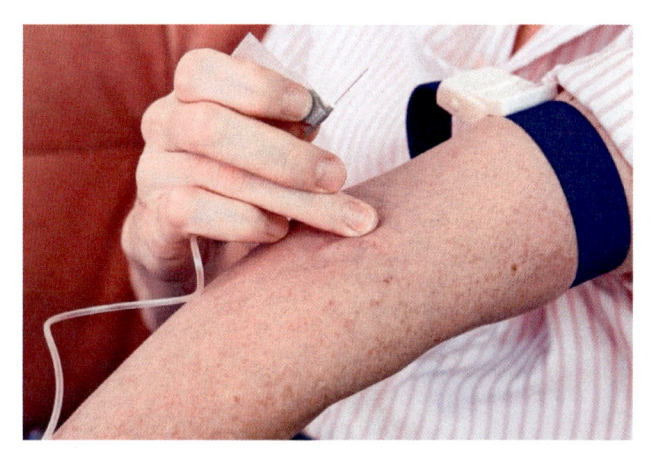

Step 13.35.
Palpate the vein.

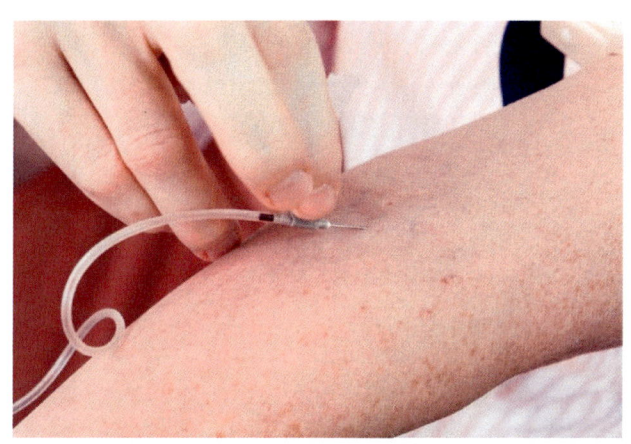

Step 13.36.
Keep the needle at 15 to 20 degrees and inject. See the blood flashback in the butterfly line. If there is no blood, do NOT proceed.

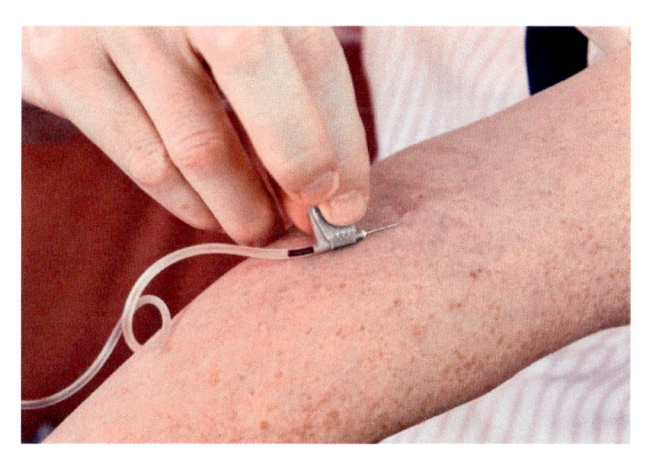

Step 13.37.
Flatten the needle against the skin.

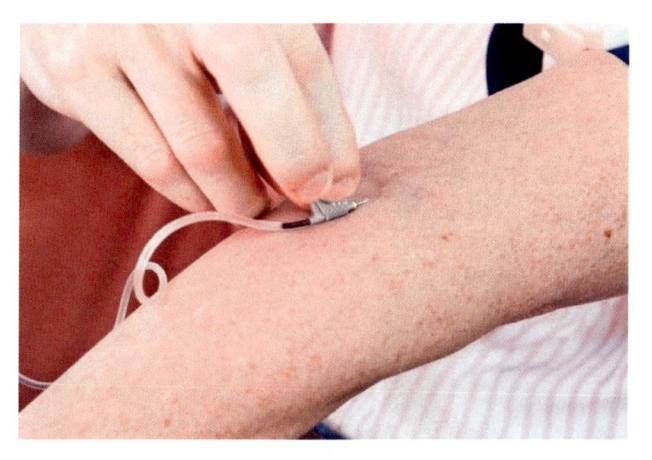

Step 13.38.
Push the needle in.

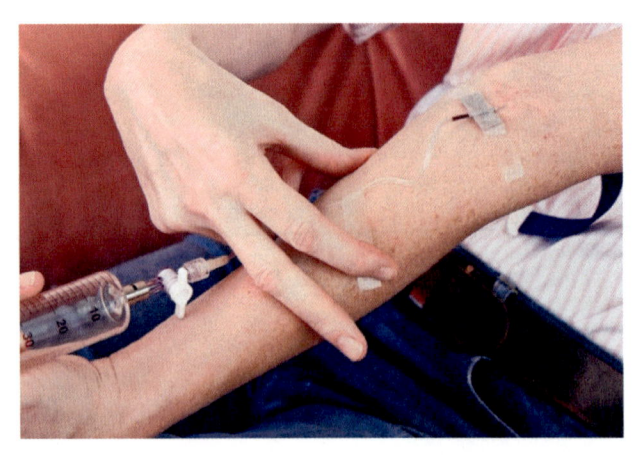

Step 13.39.
Take the second piece of tape, and tape it over the butterfly line to prevent the needle from being accidentally yanked out.

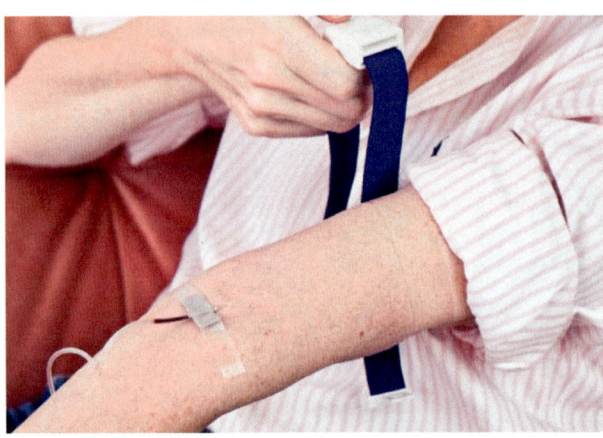

Step 13.40.
Remove the tourniquet. (VERY IMPORTANT. DO NOT FORGET!!!)

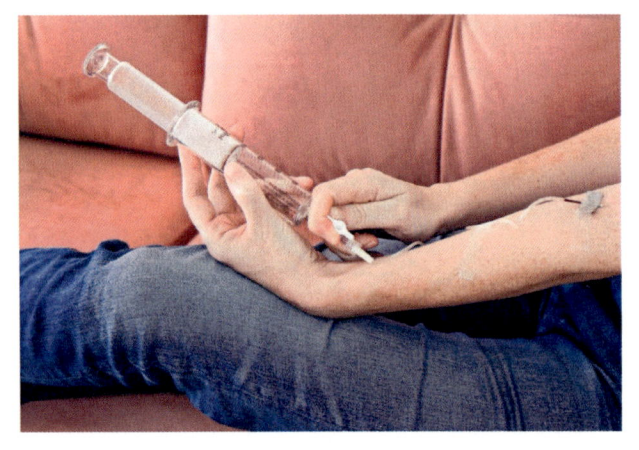

Step 13.41.
Open the ON/OFF valve attached to the syringe.

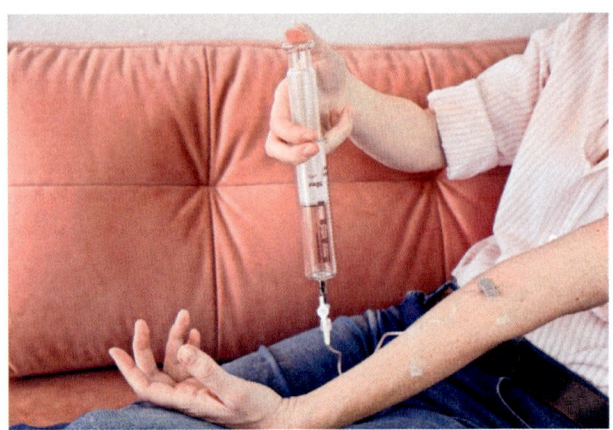

Step 13.42.
Keep the syringe upside down and keep pushing the plunger until you get the blood out of the line of the butterfly needle. Once it is out of the line, stop pushing and start counting to 20 seconds.

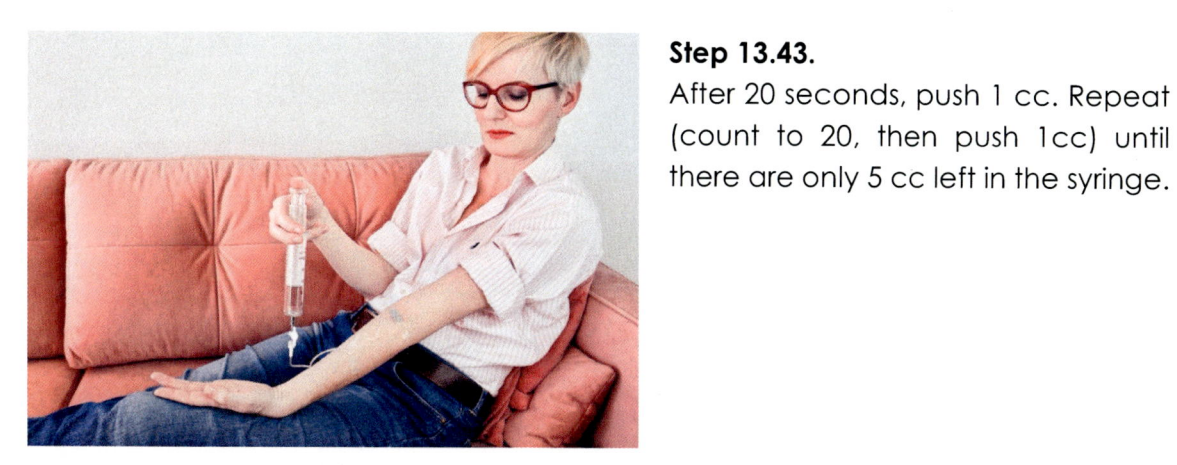

Step 13.43.
After 20 seconds, push 1 cc. Repeat (count to 20, then push 1cc) until there are only 5 cc left in the syringe.

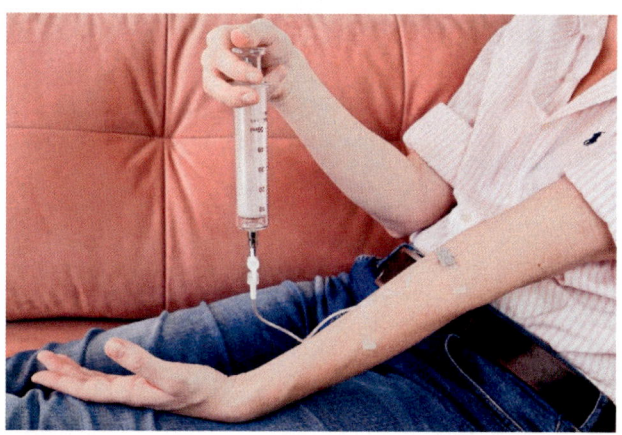

Step 13.44.
When you are down to 5 cc, you are done with the injection.

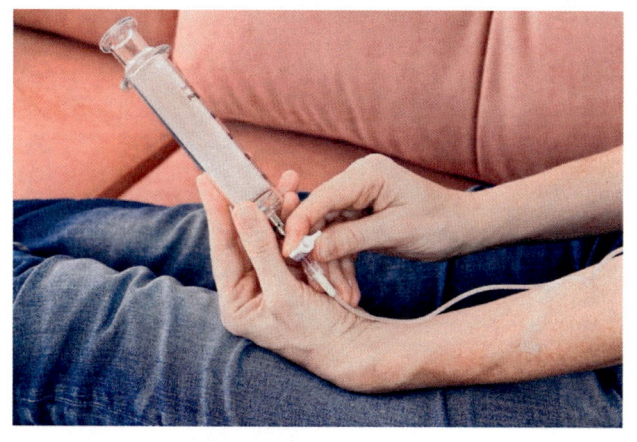

Step 13.45.
Close the ON/OFF valve. Pictures shows open, not close!

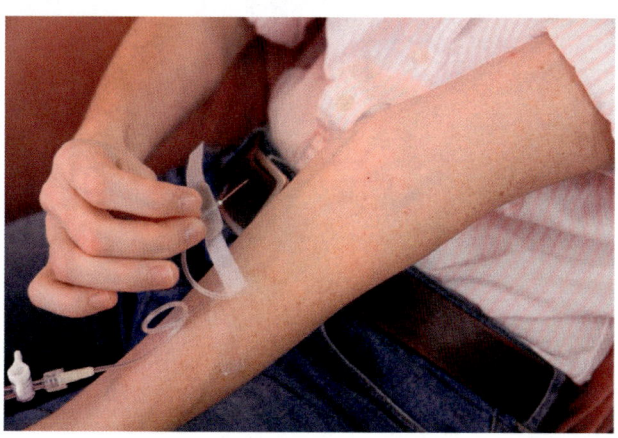

Step 13.46.
Pull out the needle. Take a cotton pad and press it down on the puncture wound for a few minutes. Put a band-aid on.

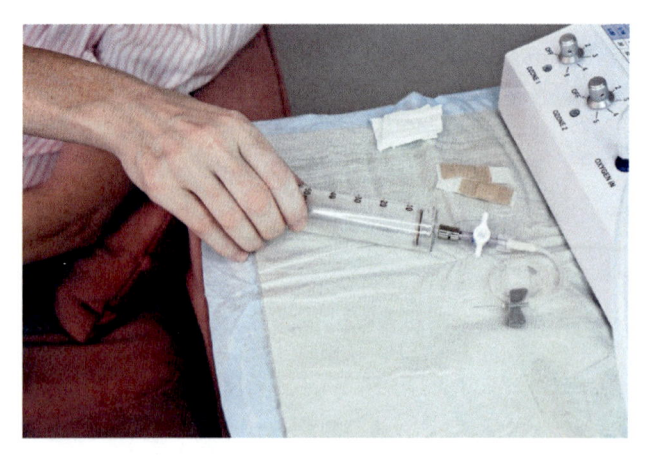

Step 13.47.
Put the syringe and needle aside. You'll take care of it later.

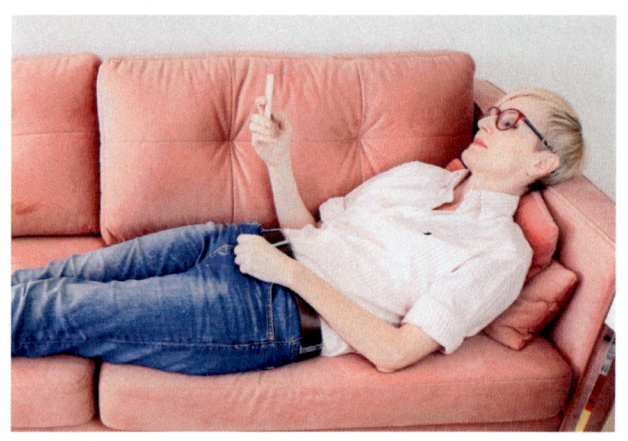

Step 13.48.
Remain reclined for at least 30 minutes. Do not move, laugh, or talk during that time.

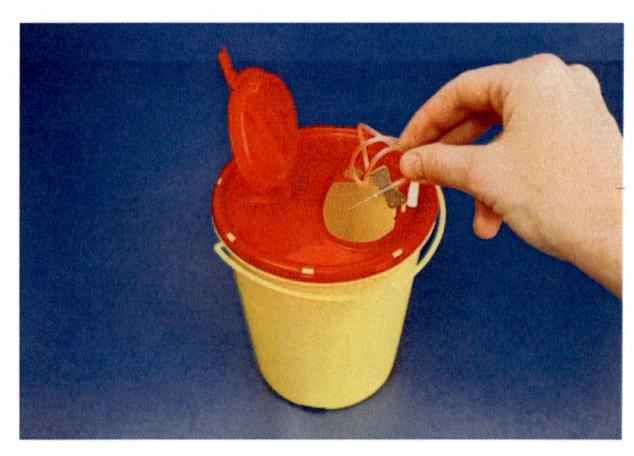

Step 13.49.
After 30 min, get up and finish everything according to steps 10.61. to 10.65.

Chapter 13 questions

1. What would happen if the two valves were set at the following position (OFF lever of the 3-way-valve turned towards the destructor and the ON/OFF valve being set to OFF) with the oxygen flowing? (see picture below)

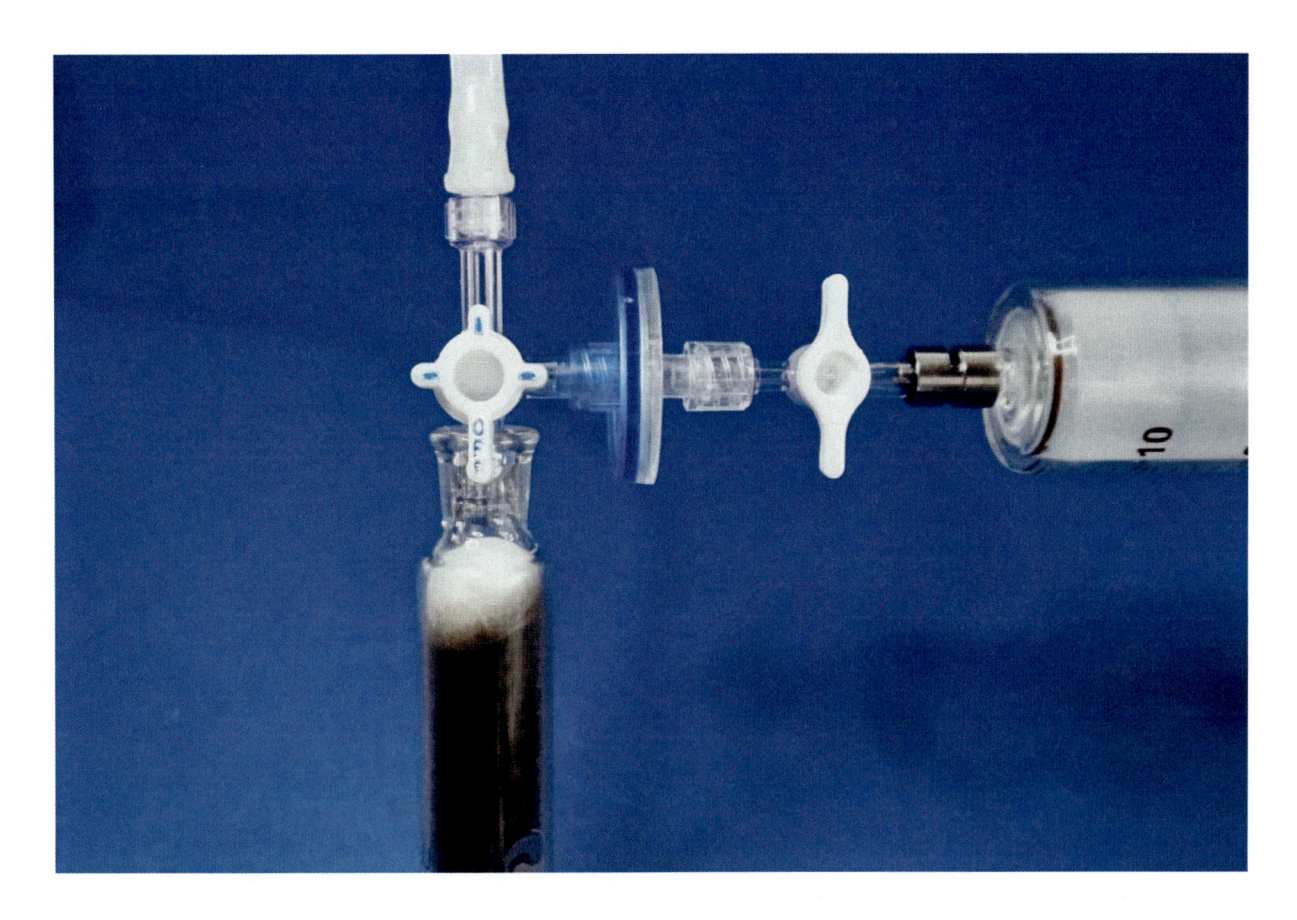

2. Why is a glass syringe not part of the "DIY for the Superparanoid" program?

3. Right after having filled the syringe, which valve do you close first? (only one correct answer)
    a) The 3-way valve of the syringe filling station
    b) The ON/OFF valve

4. What do you need to do before disconnecting the syringe from the syringe filling station? (multiple answers)
    a) Hold the syringe vertically
    b) Close the on/off valve
    c) Flush the filter with pure oxygen

5. What do you need to do if you accidentally unscrew the syringe from the ON/OFF valve instead of unscrewing the ON/OFF valve with the syringe attached to it from the filter (see picture)?

100

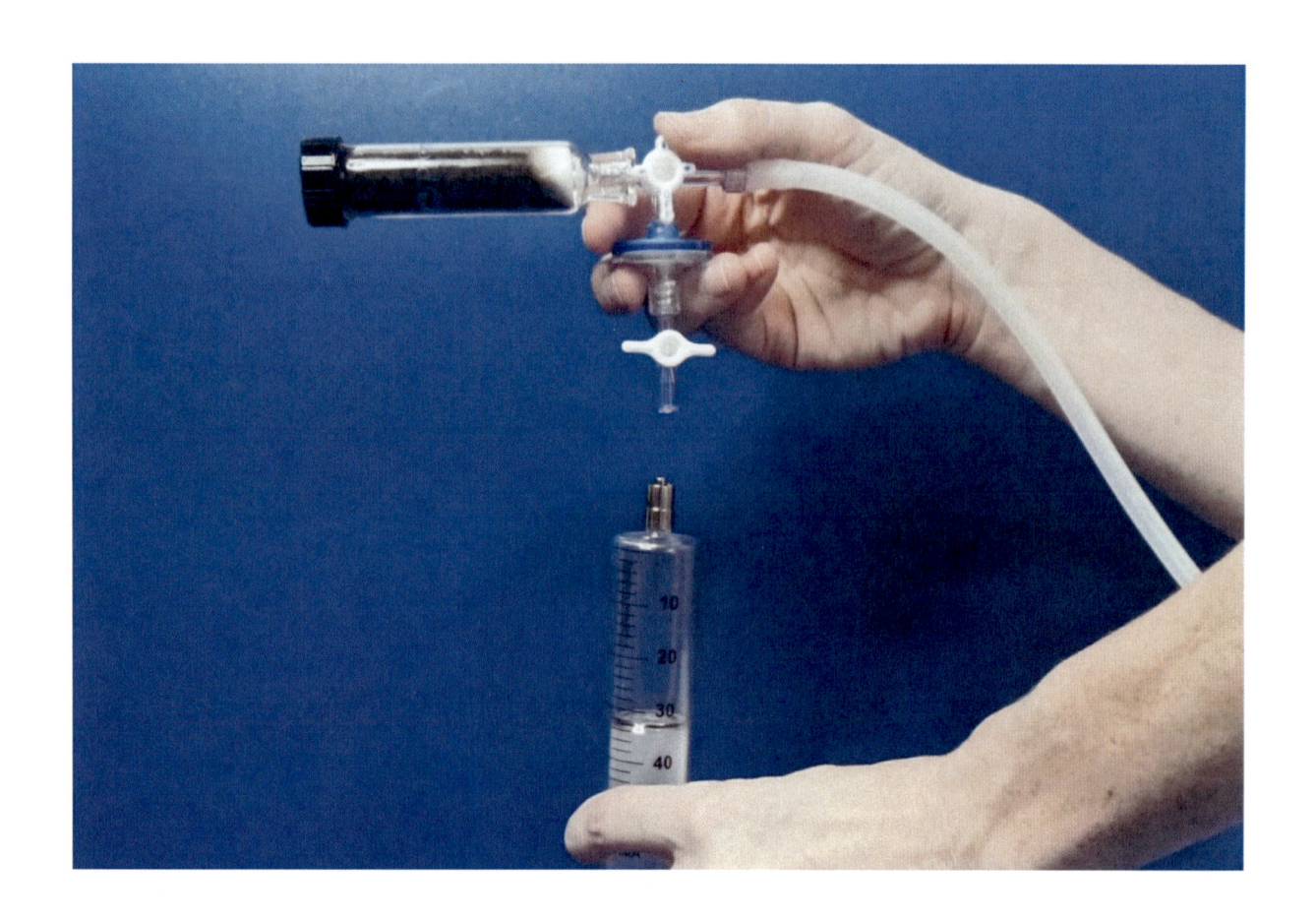

14. Troubleshooting

There are a few things which can go wrong during DIV ozone injections. Some can be fixed during the procedure, others can be remedied with supplements or ointments afterwards. The most serious complications can be prevented by following the most important precaution: **to remain horizontal and immobile for 30 minutes after the DIV.**

14.1. Chest tightness and cough

Chest tightness is the sensation of heaviness in the lungs or difficulty breathing and is a common temporary occurrence after DIV injections. It can be accompanied by a cough or harshness in the throat.

Dr. Franz Kreutzer, who wrote a book about intravenous oxygen therapy, says that the sensation of chest tightness is most likely due to micro embolisms. He assumes that intravenous oxygen injections stimulate endothelin, a peptide which causes the lung capillaries to constrict. According to his theory, this then causes the gas bubbles to get stuck and triggers the discomfort in the lungs.

Here is how to deal with it:

- **Stop the injection**: If the chest sensation sets in during the DIV, it's important to stop the procedure. Usually, the tightness disappears within 30 to 60 minutes.

- **Remain immobile**: it's important to remain horizontal, relaxed and stretched out for 30 minutes after the DIV. That's the best way to prevent it and to deal with it when it occurs.

- **Go slow**: keep at the recommended speed of 1 cc per 10 to 30 seconds. The faster you go, the more likely you will experience the lung discomfort.

- **Inject lower extremities**: the longer the path of ozone is until it reaches the lungs, the more time there is for the gas to be absorbed by the blood and the less likely the chest sensation will set in.

- **Do sports**: It appears that athletes and people who do sports regularly, exhibit the lung sensation less frequently than non-athletes. It's possible that this is because their blood has been trained to absorb more oxygen. Another possibility, as proposed by one of my clients, is that their heart ejection fraction is higher.

- **Take Theophylline**: it's a prescription medication recommended by Dr. Kreutzer, the oxyvenierung specialist. Theophylline is a vasodilator which specifically targets the small lung capillaries.

- **Drink some vitamin C**: If the lung discomfort is too strong, dissolve some vitamin C powder and drink it. Vitamin C is a powerful antioxidant and natural ozone antagonist. If taken quickly enough, it may prevent the lung sensation from getting worse. But, there is a tradeoff: it will likely cancel out some of the ozone benefits.

14.2. Trouble finding a vein

Beginners especially will have a problem with finding a vein. When starting out, it can take sometimes 5 to 6 punctures before finally seeing blood in the line of the butterfly line.

How to deal with the frustration? Keep practicing and:

- **Study the vein.** Take your time to understand how the vein runs: palpate it, get a feeling for its curves and angles. Run your finger along the vein after you apply the tourniquet. The needle should be parallel to the vein walls and not puncture through them.

- **Learn the venous puncture technique**: puncture, check for blood, flatten, and push in. Do not inject the needle through the vein. Keep an angle of around 15 to 20 degrees, puncture and then stop to check for blood flashback in the line. If there is blood, proceed, if there is no blood backflow, you're not in the vein and you need to re-adjust the needle or abort.

- **Don't give up**, keep trying. Practice makes perfect.

14.3. Blockage

Blockage is when you count to 20 and push on the plunger, just to find out that it takes much more force to get the plunger to move. You may also notice that when you release your thumb the plunger moves back to its former place. This means: nothing went in.

When this happens, there is blockage. Usually, it's because of coagulated blood in the tiny needle.

What can you do? Here are some tricks:

- Massage the spot above the injection site gently. This is sometimes enough to remove any obstruction.

- Reposition the needle. This requires some real precision work: remove the tape and change the angle of the needle without yanking it out of the vein. Move it to the right or left just a tad. You may also have to gently lift the wings of the butterfly needle to get it unstuck from to the top vein wall.

- After removing the blockage, increase the speed of the injection. It's possible you've been injecting too slowly. If you have been going at 1 cc every 20 seconds, go up to 1 cc every 15 seconds. But do not go faster than 1 cc every 10 seconds.

- Make sure you're well hydrated: drink enough water, at least 1 or 2 glasses.

- There are foods and supplements which are touted as natural blood thinners. Among them are nattokinase, green tea, ginger, turmeric and cayenne pepper. This may work only in a small percentage of people, but it may be worth a try.

How NOT to deal with blockages: do NOT use more force in the hopes of releasing the blockage through added pressure. You could succeed and as a result could push in one big chunk of gas into your vein which then could create serious problems.

14.4. Burning sensation

Burning can occur when the needle has not been inserted properly and ozone gas leaks into the surrounding tissue.

When the needle sits correctly in the vein, there should be no sensation at all (although sometimes gurgling can occur).

There are in general two different types of burning sensations:

- **Extreme burning and pain:** in this case you have no choice but to abort the injection immediately and pull the needle out.

- **Low-level burning**: you can feel that there is some irritation, but it's tolerable. You can continue with the injection in the hopes it won't get worse.

The problem with low-level burning is that it tends to escalate and become extreme, forcing you to abort the injection. So, it is better to address it early on rather than to wait. Try to gently and carefully reposition the needle just like described above under point 14.3. Change the angle by moving it slightly to the right or left or by lifting it.

14.5. Crunchiness around injection site

After the injection there can be a crunchy sensation around the puncture site. There are two different possible explanations for this:

a) Trapped oxygen gas bubbles in the vein. When pressing down along the injected vein, a crispy or crunchy sensation can be heard and felt. This is most likely due to the oxygen bubbles which have not been absorbed by the blood yet. The sensation should go away after 30 to 60 minutes. It is not dangerous. Make sure to remain immobile and horizontal during that time.

b) Oxygen gas in the tissue. If the gas did not go right into the vein but instead under the skin around the injection site, it can also result in crunchy sounds. This is also not dangerous. The gas will be absorbed within a few hours.

14.6. Allergic reaction

Some people are doubting that such a thing exists but over the years I have come across reports which allow for the strong possibility that some patients can indeed develop an allergic reaction to ozone, or to DIV injections specifically, although in my opinion this is exceedingly rare.

The signs are similar to any other allergic reaction: redness, swelling, itchiness, welt like eruptions on the skin. The reaction can be to ozone in any form or only to specific ozone applications. My Dad is fine with subcutaneous injections, ozone saunas, and breathing ozone bubbled through olive oil, but displays clear symptoms of both a systemic and local allergic reaction after DIV treatments.

If an allergic reaction after DIV occurs, discontinue the injections. Switch to other ozone applications like ozone saunas, ozone body suit, drinking ozonated water, ... etc.

In order to find out if an allergy is present, start with only small amounts of ozone/oxygen of 10 ml. If there is no adverse reaction, continue with the injections and increase the amount of ozone by 10 ml each time.

Keep in mind that ozone treatments can also trigger Herxheimer reactions. So it may be challenging to distinguish an allergic from a Herxheimer response.

14.7. Loss of consciousness

Once you lose consciousness there is not much you can do. You can only hope that when it happens you won't hurt yourself while falling down or that there is someone around who can call the ambulance.

If you live with someone, you can ask them to check on you periodically during the injection. If you live alone, you can ask a friend to watch you over Zoom during the injection.

Loss of consciousness after DIV is very rare. The most important way to prevent it is by remaining horizontal and immobile for at least 30 minutes after the injection.

In that time you should not laugh, talk, move, or get up. Just relax with your limbs stretched out for at least half an hour. Read a book or play with your smartphone. This simple precaution can prevent the most serious complications after DIV ozone treatments.

Loss of consciousness or other neurological symptoms like nausea, vomiting, confusion, memory problems, and visual disturbance are very serious complications and should be investigated carefully. The reason for any type of neurological deficit after DIV is most likely due to a gas embolism in the central nervous system.

After an fainting incidence, check the following:

- Make sure the oxygen is pure enough. Use only the recommended oxygen sources. (see chapter 5.1.)

- Do not inject too quickly. The injection speed should not be faster than 1 cc every 10 seconds and not slower than 1 cc every 30 seconds.

- Make sure that you have an air-tight oxygen circuit without leaks. With time, silicone tubing can become loose and start leaking. Check the connections regularly. If needed, exchange them for new, tighter tubing.

- Are you following all the steps? Or are you taking shortcuts? Always be conscious of what you're doing. If you're not sure if you have purged the butterfly line, abort the injection and start anew.

- Check the contraindications: are you sure none of them apply to you? If you are not sure, consult with your doctor.

Chapter 14 questions

1. What causes the chest tightness after DIV ozone injections and how can you prevent it?
2. How can you deal with a burning sensation during a DIV ozone injection?
3. How to prevent loss of consciousness?
4. What should you not do if you feel like there is a blockage?

Sources

[1] Ja-Young Jang, et al: "Nattokinase improves blood flow by inhibiting platelet aggregation and thrombus formation"
[2] Kreutzer, Franz J.: "Intravenöse Sauerstofftherapie (IOT)", 2014
[3] Annals of Pharmacotherapy, "Probable Antagonism of Warfarin by Green Tea", 1999
[4] www.healthyandnaturalworld.com: "Natural Blood Thinners: Proven Foods, Supplements and Vitamins to Thin Blood (Evidence Based)"

15. Things you should never do

Many people who practice DIV ozone injections have never received proper training in what is or what is not allowed during a venipuncture. Others get creative and try experimenting or copy what they've seen on Youtube, which can lead to disaster.

So, let's cover the biggest No No's one by one:

15.1. Do NOT get up too early
This point can't be stressed clearly enough. Most serious accidents after DIV can be avoided by heeding this one recommendation.

Remain horizontal and immobile for at least 30 min after the injection. Do not move, laugh, or conduct lively conversations during that time. Just remain relaxed, calm, and stretched out. Allow the oxygen to be fully absorbed before you get up.

I know that some doctors have their patients go and walk within minutes after DIV.

Do NOT do this.

My advice is based on the recommendations taught to oxyvenierung therapists. This is the practice of injecting pure oxygen intravenously which has been used for 60 years in Germany without a single serious complication. Why? Because oxyvenierung therapists follow this one crucial step.

15.2. Do NOT perform the injection while standing up
There are videos on Youtube showing people doing DIV ozone injections while standing, walking around, or talking.

Do NOT do this.

This can go well for some, but in others it can result in a disaster. Don't try to find out which group you belong to. You absolutely need to be in a reclined position for at least 30 minutes afterwards.

15.3. Do NOT inject too quickly
Do not inject faster than 1 cc per 10 seconds. If this gives you chest tightness, then you are going too fast. Slow down. Go down to 1 cc every 20 seconds. Use an app to help you with the countdown if necessary. Or place a clock in front of you.

15.4. Do NOT skip any steps
Go over the technique several times before you actually perform the injection. Do a couple of "dry runs" first. Keep the book right in front of you and go step by step before you actually inject yourself.

15.5. Do NOT put oil around the plunger of the syringe
Some of the ozone syringes can have a slow moving plunger which offers an extra resistance. Do not apply any oil to make it move more smoothly.

Do NOT ever do this.

Don't ever put oil onto anything which will go into your vein. Oils do not get absorbed by the blood and can cause embolisms. This is why oily substances like testosterone or vitamin D are never injected intravenously, but only intramuscularly.

15.6. Do NOT push through the chest tightness
Do not "tough it out" and keep pushing gas into your vein if you feel the chest sensation.

The feeling of heaviness in the lungs is most likely due to micro embolisms. This means that there are more oxygen bubbles in the blood than the body can absorb. By pushing in more gas you could exacerbate the situation and cause a severe complication.

The moment you feel the chest sensation, stop the injection completely. Pull out the needle, and try again the next day.

15.7. Do NOT reuse needles
Use new, fresh, sterile needles every time. Do not reuse them.

15.8. Do NOT be lax on hygiene
Do not do the injections under unsanitary, dusty, dirty conditions. Keep everything clean and tidy at all times. Wash your hands and disinfect them. Sterilize the puncture site on your arm before the injection. If you are injecting someone else - wear gloves. If you are practicing therapist, use single use supplies wherever possible.

15.9. Do NOT continue if you are unsure about steps taken
Let's say that you have already injected your vein, you see blood flashback in the line, and that's when you realize that you don't remember whether you purged the butterfly line or not. In that case - abort and start over.

Do NOT continue if you are not sure if you have followed all the steps correctly.

15.10. Do NOT push the plunger of the syringe with the tourniquet on

This is essentially Dr. Hans Wolff's technique, which I explained turned out to be disastrous in a few cases in Germany in the 1970's and 80's. People died because of it.

If you keep the vein closed while you're injecting the gas, you are creating a big bolus of gas. Once the tourniquet is loosened, that bolus is then catapulted by the blood pressure through the blood vessels which can cause deadly embolisms. Do not attempt to recreate Dr. Wolff's technique.

Once you have injected the vein and you are IN the vein, loosen the tourniquet before pressing the plunger.

15.11. Do NOT use 55 mcg/ml for non-varicose veins

There is no magic in the 55 mcg/ml number. It is not necessary to reach such high ozone concentration to achieve therapeutic effects for specific conditions.

But the risk of phlebitis and possible permanent damage of the veins is substantially higher. Doctors who use ozone concentrations of 25 to 35 mcg/ml also see results without taxing the veins unnecessarily.

15.12. Do NOT use oxygen if you are not sure about its purity

If you have doubts about the type of oxygen you're using and you are not sure if it's pure enough, then do not use it and pick one of the suggested options.

15.13. Do NOT do DIV if you don't feel confident

If in spite of all the precautions and instructions you are still afraid to do DIV ozone injections, then do not do them.

No one has to do DIV injections. There are always other options, like ozone saunas, drinking ozonated water, or ozone insufflations. You can also get other forms of ozone IVs at your doctor's office.

15.14. Do NOT experiment

Don't do things like trying to humidify the ozone before putting it in the syringe, or mixing it with other ingredients. Do not get creative, don't try to reinvent the wheel. Be careful, use the true and tested steps and precautions.

Chapter 15 questions

1. What is the single biggest mistake which accounts for most of the serious complications which have been recorded after DIV ozone injections?
2. Why should oil never be used to lubricate the plunger of the syringe?
3. Why is it important to inject the ozone slowly?

16. Where to buy the equipment

To make ordering as simple as possible, I put together a **TPO DIV package** where you only have to place 3 different orders to get all the supplies including already filled oxygen tanks.

Alternatively, you can also buy the oxygen locally, and the rest of the supplies online (find a list at thepowerofozone.com/DIV)

All the suggested items were selected to make it easier for you to order so that you don't have to search around. But, it does not mean that you won't be able to find similar, better, or more affordable equipment somewhere else which will work just as well.

Discount codes

Promolife offers a discount of 7% on all their ozone equipment to anyone who uses the code **TPODIV** (The third letter is an "O" as in Otto, NOT a zero.). SimplyO3 offers a discount of 10% to anyone who with the code **POWER**. Find the latest discount codes on the page https://thepowerofozone.com/discount-codes.

Once you have everything together, you can also book a one-on-one live online training with me. Go to thepowerofozone.com/DIV to be guided through the instructions. Readers of this book get a $50 discount with the following code: **DIVT50**.

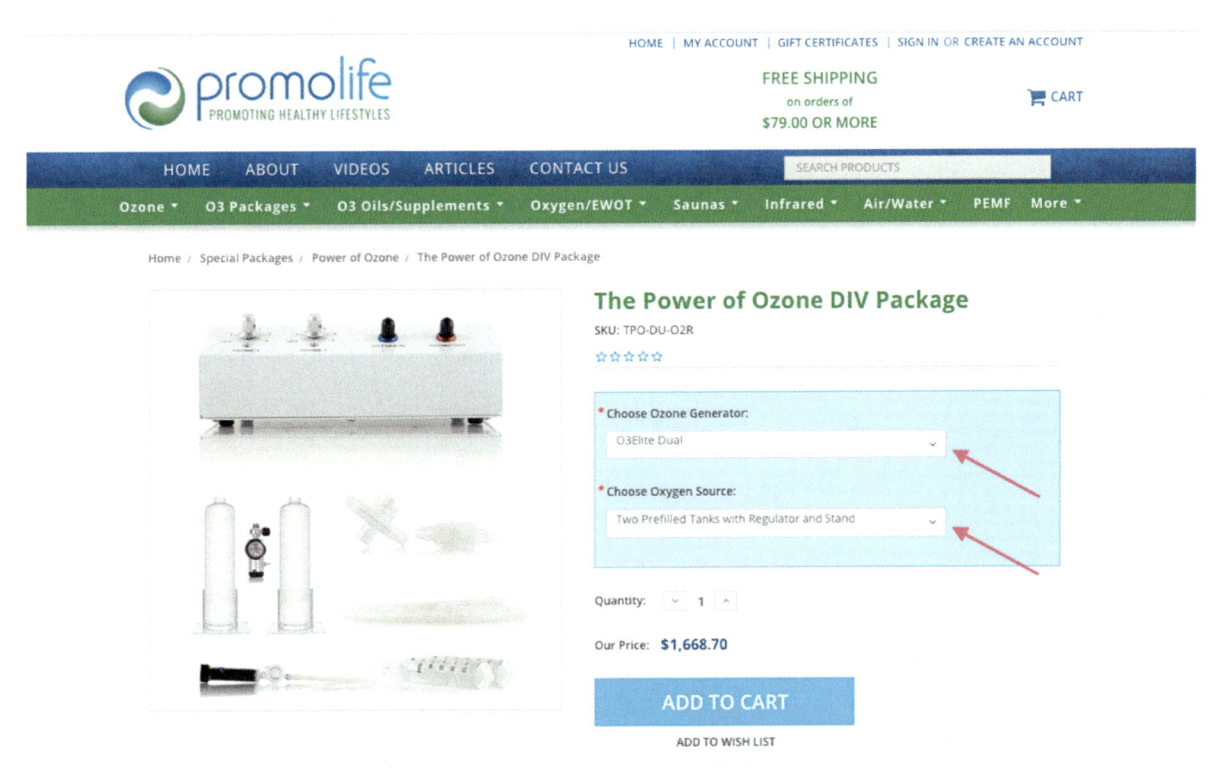

"The Power of Ozone DIV Package" from Promolife: Pick the desired ozone generator and oxygen source, or leave as is for the Dual Cell and the prefilled O2Ready tanks.

111

16.1. "The Power of Ozone DIV Package"
This is the most convenient solution. Just place the following three orders:

- Buy "The Power of Ozone DIV Package" through this link: thepowerofozone.com/DIVP, use discount code **TPODIV**
- Get 27g butterfly needles through www.medofficedirect.com
- Go to amazon.com/shop/thepowerofozone and buy everything on the "TPO DIV Supplies" list

This consists of everything you need to be able to perform DIV ozone injections: O2Ready pre-filled oxygen tanks with regulator and stand, Promolife ozone generator of your choosing, syringe filling station, extra filter, syringes, silicone tubing, luer locks, gauze, alcohol wipes, tourniquet, tape, caps, bandaids, sharps bin, butterfly needles.

When ordering the TPO DIV package you will be able to choose from five different ozone generators. My personal favorite is the **Promolife Dual Cell**, but you can pick any of the other machines.

If you prefer to shop around and buy everything separately, here are the options (don't forget to use the discount codes where applicable):

16.2. Oxygen tanks and regulators

a) Medical oxygen
Omssupply.com currently sells medical oxygen without requiring a prescription. They ship the bottles to any address in the contiguous USA and Canada, which excludes Hawaii and Alaska. A CGA 870 oxygen tank with a straight post filled with 680 L of medical oxygen currently costs US$ 125. A refill runs at US$ 35.

Important: Do NOT buy the regulator from omssupply.com. The regulator needs to be a low flow or pediatric one, which you need to buy separately, see below.

If you live in the New York City area, you can also obtain a filled medical oxygen tank without a prescription at GL Medical Equipment & Supplies in Brooklyn for US$ 99. Call in advance to check for availability.

Tanks with a straight post will require a special cylinder wrench to open.

Medical oxygen regulator
Good quality CGA 870 low flow regulators can be obtained at Promolife, SimplyO3.

Note about SimplyO3: if you own the SimplyO3 Stratus 3.0 ozone generator, it will require a special medical regulator which you can only get at SimplyO3.

Wrench
Medical tanks with a straight post (instead of a toggle) require a wrench to open.

b) Ultra high purity scientific grade oxygen

This type of oxygen can be acquired at Airgas in different sizes. An 80 CF (2,300 L) bottle costs around $330, a refill around $150. Smaller sizes may be available as well. The tanks are for pickup only.

The ultra-high purity tanks require a CGA 540 low flow regulator which is available from Promolife or SimplyO3.

Note about SimplyO3: if you own the SimplyO3 Stratus 3.0 ozone generator, it will require a special CGA 540 industrial regulator with extra flows.

c) Promolife's O2Ready pre-filled oxygen tanks

The O2Ready tanks come in pairs and can be acquired through promolife.com. Make sure that you include the special regulator with your first order.

16.3. Ozone generators

You can use any of the following machines for DIV ozone injections:

Promolife Mini
Promolife O3Elite Single
Promolife O3Elite Dual Cell (my favorite)
Promolife O3Arc Standard
Promolife O3Arc Pro

SimplyO3 Stratus 2.0
SimplyO3 Stratus 3.0
SimplyO3 Cumulus
Ozonette

Longevity EXT50
Longevity EXT120
Longevity EXT120T-Ultra
Longevity Quantum 3
Longevity Quantum 5

(For Longevity: Mention **The Power of Ozone** or my name, Paola Dziwetzki, when you place the order. Thank you!)

You can also use any Herrmann, Zotzmann, Hänsler, Kastner, Ozonosan, or Sedecal ozone machine.

A note about Longevity generators: when you place your order, make sure to ask that the quick connectors inside the tubing are exchanged for luer lock connectors. You don't want to have to do this yourself.

16.4. Supplies

You will find this list with hyperlinks to the online stores on the following website: thepowerofozone.com/DIV. Some of the supplies can be also acquired at your local pharmacy or drugstore.

- Ozone resistant syringes are sold by promolife.com and simplyO3.com
- Syringe filling station (Promolife and SimplyO3)
- Glass syringes (not part of the "DIV for the Superparanoid" method) are available at promolife.com
- Exel butterfly infusion set, 27 x ¾ inch needle, 12 inch tubing.
- Syringe filter, 0.2 um.
- Silicone tubing OD 5/16" x ID 3/16", [OD 0.8 cm x ID 0,5 cm]
- Luer lock connectors
- Sterile syringe caps
- Alcohol wipes
- Tourniquet
- Tape, transparent, 0.5 inches [ca. 1 cm] wide
- Bandaid
- Sharps bin
- Book, tablet, or smartphone

Chapter 16 questions

1. If you buy the medical oxygen from omssupply.com why do you need to buy the regulator separately?

17. How to use DIV therapeutically

Because of DIV's controversial nature and lack of research on the subject, there are no generally accepted recommendations how different conditions should be treated. Each doctor may have his or her own best approach. There is not one best ozone concentration or treatment frequency which works best for Lyme, EBV, or cancer when using intravenous ozone injections.

So, regard the following as very subjective, loose guidelines.

General recommendations

Use ozone concentrations of 20 to 35 mcg/ml for all systemic treatments.

Start with 10 cc and observe if there are signs of an allergic reaction or other troubling side effects. If there are none, continue and increase by 10 cc with each injection until you reach 60 cc. You can go above that, as long as there is no chest tightness. With the first sign of the lung sensation, stop the injection.

For a therapeutic effect, plan a minimum of 2 to 3 injections per week. The more often DIVs are performed, the faster the recovery tends to occur.

For preventive measures, do at least one injection per week.

Do not put all your eggs in one basket, always have a plan B in case of collapsed veins or other side effects.

Even the best developed veins will eventually sclerose and get damaged if they are punctured too often. This is not unique to ozone injections, but applies to all types of intravenous treatments, see people who abuse drugs.

When administering DIV ozone injections and other ozone treatments regularly, I recommend supplementing with vitamin C, since it has been found that ozone can reduce the levels of ascorbic acid in the bloodstream. If you want to preserve the maximum effect of the ozone treatment, it's suggested to space apart the ingestion of vitamin C by several hours.

DIV for infections

Ozone can be used to successfully treat a wide variety of infections. From influenza, to colds, or Lyme disease. There are even credible reports of successful Ebola treatments with DIV ozone injections.

To eliminate acute infections, intensive DIV courses should be performed. A single course can last from days to a few months, depending on the type of infection. In that time the DIVs should be performed at least 2 to 3 times a week, ideally every day. To keep veins healthy, please refer to chapter 9.4.

Once the infection has resolved completely, the ozone applications can be discontinued without the need for maintenance treatments.

During an intensive ozone course, the following pattern can be observed: After the first DIV, there is often an immediate improvement, which can vary from very mild to a near complete resolution of symptoms. If after this initial response (which can last from half an hour to several days) symptoms start creeping back in, the ozone treatments should be repeated until all symptoms have resolved and until the improvements are permanent.

The same approach can be used with chronic infections, although the process can take considerably longer.

To maximize the effect of the DIV ozone treatments, I recommend to follow a low carb, meat-based diet to keep the blood sugar low. Elevated blood glucose feeds pathogens and impairs the immune system. Especially viral infections appear to react significantly to blood sugar changes. Herpes outbreaks for example can be often controlled with a low carb diet alone.

If you go super low carb, make sure to supplement with vitamin C, since repeated high doses of ozone can reduce the vitamin C levels in our blood.

DIV for auto-immune conditions

Conditions like psoriasis, arthritis, diabetes, or lupus can be successfully treated with various types of ozone therapy including DIV ozone injections.

In those cases, ozone tends to work more as a symptom management tool than a cure. Consequently, auto-immune conditions require a long term approach during which ozone treatments have to be performed regularly. Here as well, it is highly advisable to combine ozone treatments with a sugar free, gluten free, low carb meat based diet. There are many reports of complete resolutions of auto-immune conditions with dietary changes alone.

Combining an anti-inflammatory meat based diet with ozone therapy can speed up the recovery.

The DIV ozone injections should be performed at least 2 to 3 times a week and can be combined with drinking ozonated water, ozone saunas, ozone body bag treatments, or insufflations.

DIV for treating varicose veins

The treatment of varicose veins with DIV ozone injections calls for relatively high ozone concentrations of 50 to 70 mcg/ml.

The injection will trigger phlebitis, or inflammation of the vein. This can last several days and be quite painful, especially upon walking.

Once the inflammation has resolved, the vein will have lost its discoloration and bulging. Often, a single injection will have lasting effects of up to several years. Should the bulging re-appear the injection can be repeated as often as needed.

DIV for treating cancer

Why would one want to treat cancer with ozone therapy? Because, it is possible that it works similarly to what chemotherapy and radiation does: by producing ROS, reactive oxygen species.

Current research shows that cancer cells tend to have higher ROS (reactive oxygen species) levels than healthy cells. Chemotherapy and radiation further increase the ROS to the point of pushing them over a threshold where cell death occurs.

Theoretically at least, ozone therapy could achieve the same effect without damaging healthy cells and without the risk of creating secondary cancers as is observed with chemo or radiation.

But, besides a few anecdotal cases, there are no studies which support this theory. Although, as Dr. Perez Olmedo, a Spanish oncologist, pointed out, no study has seriously tried to find out if ozone therapy could be a viable anti-cancer treatment or not.

It's understandable though if some try to look into alternative treatments, given that chemotherapy has been found to improve the 5 year survival rate on average by 2.6% (with some cancers it has been shown to contribute 0% to the survival rate; for testicular cancer it's 40%) and given that a course of chemotherapy can be grueling.

What would be the best approach if one wanted to give ozone therapy a chance? It appears that the best results can be obtained if the tumor is targeted with the ozone as directly as possible.

Example: for breast cancer, it is best to inject ozone subcutaneously in and around the tumor, cup over it with ozone (best while in the sauna), and do vaginal insufflations (because of an assumed lymphatic connection).

For prostate cancer, rectal insufflations would bring the ozone closest to the tumor and hence be the most promising ozone treatment. Together with direct ozone injections into the gland.

For lung cancer: BOOO (breathing ozonated olive oil) and ozone saunas with ozone cupping over the lungs could be the most effective.

DIV can be given as an adjunct general treatment to boost the immune system and to improve the outcome of the local ozone approaches.

For system-wide cancers like leukemia, lymphoma, or myeloma, DIV and ozone saunas could be the best approach.

DIV as a preventive measure

It is difficult to devise a concrete protocol for those who wish to do DIV ozone treatments only as a prophylactic. If there are no health problems present, then it's hard to tell whether what one is doing works or not.

In general, doing DIV ozone injections at least once per week is probably enough to maintain a good status quo.

Chapter 17 questions

1. What is the difference in approach when treating an acute infection versus an auto-immune condition with DIV ozone injections?
2. What type of a diet can optimize the outcomes of ozone treatments?
3. Why is it a good idea to have a backup plan when undergoing DIV ozone injections?
4. What is the rationale behind why ozone therapy could be a potentially effective cancer treatment?

Sources
[1] Rowen, Robert J.: "Rapid Resolution of Hemorrhagic fever (Ebola) in Sierra Leone With Ozone Therapy"
[2] American Addiction Editorial Staff: "Collapsed Veins Due to IV Drug Use"
[3] Sanchez, Albert, et al: "Role of sugars in human neutrophilic phagocytosis"
[4] Science Daily: "High blood sugar of diabetes can cause immune system malfunction, triggering infection"
[5] Kazue Takahashi: "Dietary sugars inhibit biologic functions of the pattern recognition molecule, mannose-binding lectin"
[6] meatrx.com, success stories

[7] Renate Viebahn-Hänsler: "Ozon-Sauerstoff-Therapie", 2009

[8] Dr. Perez Olmedo: "La Ozonoterapia, terapia complementaria. Debe ser obligatoria en el tratamiento del cáncer. Caerán de la burra. Llegará."

[9] Haotian Yang, et al: "The role of cellular reactive oxygen species in cancer chemotherapy", 2018

[10] Paola Dziwetyki: "116 REPORTS OF CANCER SUCCESSFULLY TREATED WITH OZONE THERAPY*", 2016

[11] American Cancer Society, cancer.org: "Second Cancers Related to Treatment"

[12] Graeme Morgan: "The Contribution of Cytotoxic Chemotherapy to 5-year Survival in Adult Malignancies", 2004

[13] Bocci, Velio: "Ozone, a New Medical Drug", 2005

[14] Michael Wallington et al: "30-day mortality after systemic anticancer treatment for breast and lung cancer in England: a population-based, observational study", 2016

[15] Franzini, M. et al: "First Evaluations of Oxygen-Ozone Therapy in Antibiotic-Resistant Infections", 2016

[16] thepowerofozone Youtube channel: 'Judy Seeger: "How I got rid of Lyme with ozone saunas and insufflations"'

[17] thepowerofozone Youtube channel: 'Jeff: "How ozone helped me get over Lyme"'

18. How to deal with Herxheimer reactions?

When doing DIV ozone treatments, or any other form of ozone therapy, always be prepared for an ozone induced Herxheimer reaction. Sometimes also abbreviated with a "herx", this is a type of a healing crisis, also called a detox or die-off reaction.

A die-off reaction is due to endotoxins, which are released when pathogens die. These molecules can mimic symptoms of the infection while the body is getting rid of it.

Example: when undergoing ozone therapy for a lung infection which causes shortness of breath, cough, fever, and malaise, those very symptoms can temporarily get worse or re-emerge, giving the false impression that the infection is intensifying, instead of receding.

It can be confusing to attempt to distinguish a Herxheimer reaction from an adverse reaction, since there are no established clear signs how to tell one from the other.

The following are pointers which I've collected over the years and which can offer clues about what may be going on:

A Herxheimer reaction usually sets in after an initial improvement in symptoms. So right after the ozone treatment there can be a betterment, then a worsening. The worsening can be the healing crisis.

If there is a new found well-being after the worsening passes, then this is also a sign that the worsening could have been a herx.

If the worsening can be overcome (even if only temporarily) with additional ozone treatments, then this is another possible indication that one is dealing with Herx reactions.

Often observed symptoms during herxes are fatigue, increased need for sleep which tends to be very refreshing, runny nose, coughing up phlegm, rashes, fever, feeling flu-like, achy joints, achiness throughout the body. In general it can be a retracing of symptoms of the condition which is being treated or of past infections.

If the ozone therapy is continued throughout the herxes, the moments of improvement can be often prolonged and maintained until they are permanent and a new level of well-being is achieved.

How to deal with an ozone induced Herxheimer reaction?

- Continue with the ozone treatments. More ozone can resolve ozone induced Herxheimer reactions.
- Wait it out. A Herxheimer reaction can pass by itself. Expect that with every additional ozone treatment, a new herx reaction will be triggered. This can repeat itself until the pathogen is completely eradicated.

- Reduce the frequency and duration of ozone treatments and/or the ozone concentration. By scaling down the amount and/or frequency of ozone treatments, the herxes can be reduced but the whole healing process is prolonged. So it can be a trade-off.

- Take vitamin C: dissolve ascorbic acid powder in water or take liposomal vitamin C. Keep in mind that vitamin C will also negate some of the ozone effect. So, again it's a trade-off between feeling immediately better or taking advantage of the entire ozone effect.

- Drink ozonated water. Ozonate distilled or reverse osmosis filtered water and drink 1 to 4 glasses throughout the day. Drinking ozone water is an underrated treatment which can help with both an ozone induced Herx reaction as well as with many other conditions.

Chapter 18 questions

1. What is a Herxheimer reaction?
2. How to distinguish a Herxheimer reaction from an adverse reaction?
3. How to deal with a Herxheimer reaction?

Sources
[1] Wikipedia: "Jarisch–Herxheimer reaction"

19. How safe are DIV ozone injections?

As described in chapter 3 the risks associated with DIV ozone injections can be extremely serious and even lead to death. But how often do they happen and how do the risks compare to other interventions?

It appears that serious complications after DIV ozone injections are exceedingly rare. In addition, when comparing direct ozone injections with other common medical interventions like over the counter drugs or even chiropractic adjustments, remarkably, the ozone injections tend to be considerably safer.

When was the first DIV ozone injection performed?

The injection of pure oxygen intravenously dates back more than a 100 years. The first successful intravenous injection of oxygen into dogs dates back to 1811 and was performed by a Dr. Nysten. The first intravenous oxygen injection into humans has been described by Mariani in 1902.

The first injection of an intravenous ozone/oxygen mix into a human was most likely performed in the 1930s by either Dr. Payr or Dr. Bircher.

How many DIV injections are being performed safely?

Due to the controversial nature of DIV ozone injections, many practitioners refuse to disclose whether they're performing this treatment so we don't have exact numbers how often, by whom, and where DIV injections are done.

Apart from one person in the field, statistics on DIV treatments are not collected in any kind of systematic way. So, the following information is based on estimations and guesses from selected sources:

Dr. Howard Robins, one of the most prolific DIV practitioners, claims to have performed over 310,000 DIV ozone injections without a single fatality.

(Note: In 2019, Dr. Robins was sued by a former patient for causing harm in the form of severe neurological symptoms like paralysis, memory loss, chronic fatigue, and personality changes which required hospitalization. Dr. Robins maintains that the patient did not experience any long term damage and that the lawsuit is frivolous. The lawsuit has been dismissed by the NY Supreme Court. The decision has been appealed by Dr. Robins' accuser and is awaiting a new decision.)

Although it's not his preferred ozone method, Dr. Robert Rowen has been performing DIVs since the 1980's. He also co-authored a paper about his and Dr. Robins' work in Africa on Ebola patients who were treated with, among others, DIV ozone injections. Dr. Rowen has also been supporting the use of DIV during the Coronavirus outbreak.

Dr. Olmedo in Spain, an oncologist, has been an ardent supporter and enthusiastic practitioner of ozone therapy, including DIV ozone injections and has published several Facebook posts extolling the benefits of DIV injections.

A local "underground" practitioner in New Jersey has been performing DIV ozone injections for the past 30 years. I estimate that the number of infusions he has done in that time lies at roughly 30,000, probably more. When I used to visit him more than 10 years ago, there was always a queue of at least 2 or 3 people in his office, so the above number is a very conservative estimate.

There is also an individual who does the same on the West Coast who has been practicing for over 20 years. According to his own calculations, he must have also performed around 30,000 DIVs by now.

A doctor in Columbia has been performing DIV ozone injections in his practice for years. A few members of the Facebook "The Ozone Group" traveled all the way to South America to receive 10 pass treatments and DIV ozone injections at the hands of the medic.

Another practitioner in Mexico has been applying this method for the past 5 to 6 years, and at an increased rate during Corona times. He estimates that he has done around 1,000 DIVs.

Those are just a few examples of doctors who practice DIV. The total number of practitioners who use this method safely without causing any casualties may be in the hundreds or thousands worldwide.

Which means that thousands of DIVs are being performed every year all around the world, in most cases without any major incidents.

In addition there is the art of oxyvenierung which has been practiced in Germany for the past 60 years. Although it is not ozone therapy, it is very similar to DIV: it's the injection of pure oxygen intravenously.

During a conversation with a representative of the Oxyven company (the manufacturer of the oxyvenierung machines), I was told that based on their inventory a total of 100,000 to 150,000 intravenous oxygen treatments must be performed every year.

This means that in the past 60 years, an estimated 3 to 4 million intravenous oxygen injections have been executed in one country alone, without a single fatality.

During the same time, probably a few million DIV ozone injections must have been performed. This makes the two different types of intravenous oxygen injections some of the safest medical interventions in existence, as long as they are being performed correctly.

How does the risk from DIV ozone injections compare with other interventions?

Yes, DIV ozone injections, especially when performed incorrectly, can cause some very serious side-effects including death. But so do over the counter drugs, chiropractic adjustments, or simply drinking water.

A cursory search produced 19 well-documented cases of people having died from drinking water in the past 30 years. That's more than from any type of ozone therapy in the same time period.

A review from 2010 listed 26 well documented cases of death after chiropractic adjustments. That's 4 times more than what has been reported from DIV so far. Given that chiropractic has become more popular and has even gained the approval of the FDA, it can be assumed that the number of fatalities from structural manipulations has only grown since.

Between 150 and 500 people die each year in the US due to Tylenol, an over the counter medication. At least 7,600 people die every year due to non-steroidal anti-inflammatory drugs (NSAIDs) like aspirin, another over the counter drug.

Which means that in the last 20 years those two medications have killed at least 155,000 more Americans than ozone therapy.

But of course all of this pales in comparison to the genocide legally perpetrated every year by modern medicine: It is estimated that between 40,000 and 250,000 people die each year due to medical errors in the US alone. This does not include the around 128,000 deaths annually due to correctly taken medications.

Seen in context, DIV ozone injections, and ozone therapy in general, are one of the safest medical interventions ever devised.

Chapter 19 questions

1. How many DIVs has Dr. Robins performed in the past 30 years without causing a single death?
2. Around how many Oxyvenierung treatments (intravenous oxygen) have been performed in Germany in the past 60 years without a single death?
3. How many documented cases are there which show people having died due to water intoxication?
4. How many Americans die due to Tylenol and Aspirin every year?

Sources

[1] Paola Dziwetzki: "Can DIV ozone injections lead to death?", 2020
[2] Facebook chat with Dr. Howard Robins' associate
[3] Rowen et al,: "Rapid resolution of hemorrhagic fever (Ebola) in Sierra Leone with ozone therapy", 2016
[4] Paola Dziwetzki: "Home Ozone Treatments for the Coronavirus Infection – How Effective Are They?"
[5] Youtube, Dr. med. Dirk Wiechert channel: "Oxyven Therapy by Dr. med. Dirk Wiechert", 2013
[6] E. Ernst: "Deaths After Chiropractic: A Review of Published Cases", 2010
[7] Zach Schonfeld, The Atlantic: "150 Americans Die Each Year from Tylenol's Most Active Ingredient", 2013
[8] Laura Donnelly, The Telegraph: "Daily aspirin behind more than 3,000 deaths a year, study suggests", 2017
[9] Linda T. Kohn et al: "To Err Is Human: Building a Safer Health System", 2000
[10] John Hopkins Medicine: "Study Suggests Medical Errors Now Third Leading Cause of Death in the U.S.", 2016
[11] Michael O. Schroeder, US News: "Death By Prescription", 2016
[12] welt.de: "Triathlet (30) stirbt, weil er zu viel Wasser trank", 2015
[13] This document mentions a total of 17 fatalities due to drinking too much water: Hew-Butler Tamara et al: "Statement of the Third International Exercise-Associated Hyponatremia Consensus Development Conference, Carlsbad, California, 2015", 2015
[14] lastampa.it: "Beve troppa acqua e muore", 2008
[15] Geoffrey Bourne, and Ralph G. Smith: "The value of intravenous and intraperitoneal administration of oxygen", 1927
[16] Justia US Law: "Georgievski v Robins"
[17] J.F. Fries: "Assessing and Understanding Patient Risk", 1992
[18] Scheel, Paul: "Die Transfusion des Blutes und Einsprützung der Arzneyen in die Adern. Historisch und in Rücksicht auf die practische Heilkunde bearbeitet", 1828
[19] Cole, Frank: "Intravenous Oxygen", 1950
[20] Damiani, E. et al: "Exploring alternative routes for oxygen administration", 2016

20. Answers

Chapter 2 answers

1. DIV ozone injections describe a medical procedure during which pure ozone/oxygen gas is slowly injected intravenously at 1 cc every 10 to 30 seconds with a 27g butterfly needle.

2. The "DIV for the Superparanoid" method allows to gain confidence through paranoia since it's based on hypothetical worst case scenarios and devises methods to proactively prevent them.

3. The four tenets upon which the safety of the "DIV for the Superparanoid" method hinges upon, are:

    1. Ozone is heavier than air.
    2. Gas embolisms are mostly caused by air, not pure oxygen.
    3. It can take a while for oxygen to be absorbed by the blood cells, it's not always an instantaneous process.
    4. Gas trapped in the blood circulation rises to the highest point in the body, the brain.

4. The two main reasons why it's important to remain immobile for at least 30 minutes after a DIV ozone injection are:

    a. It takes a while for the oxygen to be absorbed by the red blood cells. It's assumed that this can take between 20 to 40 minutes.
    b. During this time, the body should be placed in a horizontal position, since gas which is trapped inside the blood circulation will rise to the highest point, the brain.

Chapter 3 answers

1. Known cases of death after DIV ozone injections occurred in Germany in the 1970's and 1980's. A total of six cases have been reported in that time after various ozone therapy treatments, three of which were confirmed to be after DIV ozone injections. The remaining three were after a subcutaneous injection around a leg ulcer, one was after an intra-arterial injection, and the other occurred 3 weeks after a DIV procedure with the official cause of death being listed as pneumonia.

Another was reported in Las Vegas where two men met with two women in a private apartment where something called "octozone" was performed. One of the women lost consciousness and perished a week later at a hospital.

2. Dr. Hans Wolff's method consisted of binding off the vein of the patient as long as the gas was being injected and leaving the tourniquet in place for up to 20 min. Once the tourniquet was removed, the patient was allowed to get up.

   What made Dr. Wolff's technique dangerous, was
   that it must have led to a bolus of gas being catapulted through the blood vessels the moment the tourniquet was released. This must have resulted in the gas entering the arterial circulation (in patients with a possible ventricular septal defect) and causing fatal embolisms in the brain.

   Dr. Wolff was not respecting the most important tenets: to inject the gas slowly, to wait 30 minutes after the injection to allow the gas to be absorbed (without the applied tourniquet), and the fact that gas in the blood will rise to the highest point, the brain.

3. The chest tightness is most likely due to two factors: the production of endothelin, a peptide which causes the narrowing of lung capillaries in the lungs, and the presence of oxygen bubbles. Those two things together cause micro embolisms in the lungs, something which is also observed during oxyvenierung, or the intravenous injection of pure oxygen.

4. The following neurological symptoms could be an indication that a gas embolism has occurred in the brain: memory loss, confusion, dizziness, speech impediment, paralysis, loss of consciousness, visual disturbance.

Chapter 4 answers

1. The known contraindications for ozone therapy are: ventricular septal defect, hyperthyroidism (which is not well controlled through medication), medical emergencies (like heart attack, stroke, physical trauma, asthma attack, bleeding), transplanted organs, allergic reaction, and phlebitis.

   The theoretical contraindications are G6PD deficiency, or eosinophilia.

   People who have difficulty following instructions, should
   also abstain from performing DIV ozone injections.

2. Ozone treatments can stimulate the immune system. People with transplanted organs have to take immune suppressing medication to make sure that their immune system does not refuse the foreign organ. Ozone therapy works exactly in the opposite fashion: it boosts the immune system, so ozone treatments could lead to the rejection of a transplanted organ.

3. A ventricular septal defect could lead to oxygen/ozone gas entering the arterial circulation. This could then lead to a gas embolism in the central nervous system.

Chapter 5 answers

1. Oxygen used for DIV ozone injections has to be at least 99% pure.

2. No, it can't. The syringe filling station is central to the "DIV for the Superparanoid" method. Alternatively, a syringe filling station can be also made out of a destructor system, a three-way-valve, a luer lock connector pair, a piece of silicone tubing, and a filter.

3. For DIV ozone injections either 27g or 25g butterfly needles can be used, but not bigger. The tiny diameter of the needle makes sure that the created oxygen bubbles are as small as possible which is central to maintain the safety of the protocol.

4. To ascertain the utmost cleanliness during DIV ozone injections, the following supplies are used:

    - a new, sterile butterfly needle
    - alcohol wipes to clean the puncture site, the syringe, and the filter
    - a sterile syringe cap to close the filter and the syringe after the injection to protect them from dust and dirt.
    - a new, sterile syringe for each patient (when used by a practitioner), and also a new, sterile filter.

5. Used needles need to be tossed either into a sharps bin or into an empty detergent bottle. When the bin is full, it is closed and thrown into the garbage. This is done to protect whoever will pick the garbage, be it a family member, or the garbage collector. The bin protects them from being punctured and potentially infected by the used needles.

6. The tape should be either 0.5" wide (ca. 1 cm) or transparent to make sure that it does not obscure the view on the butterfly line to check for blood flashback.

7. The syringe caps prevent dust and dirt from entering the filter and the syringe.

Chapter 6 answers

1. The tape, cotton pads, and band-aid should be at arm's length from where you will perform the injection, so that you can grab them without having to get up. Immediately after the injection you are not allowed to rise and need to remain horizontal and immobile for at least 30 minutes. Keeping the supplies at arm's length allows you to grab them without having to change your reclined position.

2. In order to keep everything as clean and sterile as possible, you should

    - clean and disinfect your hands
    - clean the surface area
    - use an underpad for the working station
    - disinfect the filter and syringe with an alcohol wipe
    - use sterile supplies as much as possible: the butterfly needle, and if you're treating patients also the filter and the syringe
    - use sterile caps for the filter and the syringe after the DIV (if they will be re-used)

3. It is important to wear loose clothes during DIV injections since tight clothes could impair blood circulation. Clothes which cut into armpits or the groin area (if the legs or feet are injected) could prevent blood from flowing freely. Loosely fitting garments prevent larger gas bubbles from forming which could create complications when released with a sudden move.

4. You should carve out around 1 hour for DIV ozone injections. The preparation alone can take around 5 to 10 minutes and you need to remain horizontal and immobile for at least 30 minutes afterwards. That's 35 to 45 minutes. Also allow some extra time in case you won't find the vein right away and need to restart the whole process.

    During that time you want to make sure to be undisturbed to prevent a situation where you may have to jump up to open the door right after you finished the DIV. This could trigger a severe chest tightness sensation and even lead to loss of consciousness or worse (see chapter 3).

Chapter 7 answers

1. The two main tools to create an air-tight oxygen circuit are: a) tightly fitting silicone tubing, b) luer lock connectors.

2. If silicone tubing is attached to luer locks and other connectors for too long it can become deformed and loose. This can lead to leaks. For this reason, the attachments between connectors and silicone tubing should be regularly checked and if they have become unreliable, they should be exchanged for new tubing.

3. PVC tubing should not be used to connect the oxygen source with the ozone generator since it does not create as tight of a connection with luer locks and other connectors as silicone tubing. A loose connection could cause gas leaks.

Chapter 8 answers

1. Oxygen tanks require special attention because they contain highly pressurised contents. If a tank is grossly mishandled, it could turn into a missile and do great damage to humans and property.

2. The correct way to open a tank is by turning the valve only halfway. The correct way to close it is by not exerting too much force on the valve in order to not damage the seal.

3. An oxygen tank should be kept out of the sun and away from other heat sources to prevent the gas from expanding and the valve from bursting.

Chapter 9 answers

1. Yes, varicose veins can be used to perform DIV ozone injections. If the ozone concentration is high enough, this can result in the veins losing their bulging and discoloration.

2. The needle should always be injected in the direction of the flow of the blood, towards the heart.

3. The problem with veins around the wrist is that although they are often prominent and well defined, they tend to roll and move when injected.

4. Use the following two tricks to fixate a rolling vein: a) apply two tourniquets close to each other to fixate the vein, b) stretch and fixate the vein with two fingers of your hand.

5. The best trick to make a vein fill up and plump up: lower the arm all the way down to the ground, keep pumping the fist for a minute or two, and then to put on the tourniquet.

Chapter 10 answers

1. The four tenets upon which the "DIV for the Superparanoid" method rests, are:

    A. Ozone is heavier than air.
    B. During DIV injections only pure oxygen/ozone gas mix can be injected, never air.
    C. The absorption of oxygen by the red blood cells is not an instantaneous process.
    D. Gas bubbles rise in the human body to the highest point, the brain.

2. Correct answer: b)

3. Correct answer: a)

4. The syringe port including the syringe filter has just been flushed with pure oxygen. If the filter were pointing down instead of up, the oxygen could pour out and air could enter. By keeping the filter pointing up until the syringe is screwed in it's ensured that no air will enter the filter.

5. By holding the syringe filling station up and by keeping the syringe vertically before unscrewing it, there is no need to flip it. When flipped, air could enter the syringe. No flip, no risk of getting air inside.

6. Correct answer: b)

7. It is important to not let the butterfly needle dangle, since ozone is heavier than air and it could pour out of the butterfly needle and air could enter.

Chapter 11 answers

1. When the first injection is finished, so when there are only 5 cc left inside the syringe, grab the end piece of the butterfly line and hold it up. Then, unscrew the syringe from the butterfly line. Grab the second syringe, all the while holding the end piece of the butterfly needle pointing up.

Move the syringe as close as possible to the end piece of the butterfly line, so that they touch each other. Then, with one quick move, flip the syringe upside down and screw it onto the butterfly end piece. Keep pushing the plunger at a pace of 1 cc every 10 to 30 seconds.

2. The second syringe, will be parked upright in a glass for the duration of the injection of the first syringe. This can take 10 to 20 minutes. During that time the ozone will start to break down inside the syringe. To account for the loss in ozone concentration, one can choose a slightly higher ozone concentration.

3. The second syringe, once filled, should be placed upright. Either by using a glass or a vial stand. This is to ensure that no ozone will pour out of the syringe since ozone is heavier than air.

Chapter 12 answers

1. The recommended ozone concentration to successfully treat varicose veins ranges from 50 to 70 mcg/ml.

2. During DIV ozone injections to treat varicose veins you should take care not to create kinks in your legs. So your limbs should be stretched out as much as possible to ensure an unhindered circulation of the blood.

3. After the injection the vein will become inflamed, red, and painful. This is phlebitis, or inflammation of the vein. It will last 3 to 4 days during which walking can become quite painful. Once this has resolved, the vein will have lost its bulging and discoloration.

Chapter 13 answers

1. Since the OFF button on the 3-way-valve is turned towards the destructor, the oxygen has only one way to go: towards the syringe. But the ON/OFF valve leading towards the syringe is closed. So the oxygen has no way to go. Pressure will build up which will lead to the bursting open of the weakest part in the oxygen's path: one of the connections will pop: either the silicone tubing from the regulator, or the silicone tubing around one of the luer lock connectors.

2. A glass syringe is not part of the "DIV for the Superparanoid" method since it is much more difficult to handle and it is much easier to accidentally allow air to enter.

3. Correct answer: a)

4. Correct answers: a) and b)

5. If the syringe is accidentally unscrewed from the ON/OFF valve instead of the ON/OFF valve together with the syringe from the filter, then the procedure needs to be aborted and re-started from scratch.

    The reason for this is that when the syringe alone is unscrewed (without the ON/OFF valve), the plunger likely slipped and sucked some air inside. At the same time the oxygen/ozone which was at the bottom part of the ON/OFF valve escaped and air entered.

    You may have to also buy a new syringe, since if you unscrew it without the ON/OFF valve, it's possible that the plunger will fall out and break.

Chapter 14 answers

1. The chest tightness which often occurs after and during DIV ozone injections is most likely due to micro embolisms in the lungs.

    The same phenomenon also occurs during oxyvenierung, or the injection of pure oxygen. It's assumed that it's a combination of vasoconstriction of small lung capillaries and the introduction of the gas bubbles.

    To prevent the chest tightness, inject slowly, remain horizontal and immobile during the DIV, do not to talk, do not to laugh, and do not make any lively movements for at least 30 minutes afterwards.

    When the lung discomfort occurs during the injection, the injection should be stopped immediately.

2. Burning sensation around the injection site usually indicates that there is leakage into the surrounding tissue. Which means that the needle is not positioned properly. The way to fix this is to gently adjust the needle to change its angle. It may be also necessary to lift it a bit to get it unstuck from the upper vein wall.

3. The most important way to prevent loss of consciousness after DIV ozone injections is to remain immobile and horizontal for a good 30 minutes afterwards.

4. If there is a blockage, you should never try to push through it by exerting more force. This could result in a big bolus of gas being released and catapulted through your veins which could result in a very dangerous situation.

Chapter 15 answers

1. The biggest mistake is to not rest after the ozone injection. Do not ever skip this step. Don't ever get up right after the injection. Rest for at least 30 minutes.

2. Oil should never be inside a syringe which is used to perform any type of intravenous injections. Once oil is inside the bloodstream it can cause embolisms. This is why oily substances like vitamin D, E, or testosterone are never injected intravenously but always into the muscle.

3. It is of paramount importance to inject the gas slowly since it can take a certain amount of time for the oxygen to be absorbed. It is not an instantaneous process.

Chapter 16 answer

1. The regulator which is sold with the pre-filled medical oxygen tank by omssupply.com is a high flow regulator. It can't be used with most ozone generators for personal use. The correct regulator is a so-called pediatric or low flow regulator and can be obtained from Promolife, SimplyO3, Amazon, or Longevity.

Chapter 17 answers

1. An acute infection usually calls for a single, intensive ozone course which is performed during a limited time period. Ozone can resolve the infection permanently without the need for repeat or maintenance treatments.

   An auto-immune condition on the other hand, usually can not be fully resolved with ozone. Here, ozone therapy is used more as a symptom management tool which needs to be applied regularly and possibly indefinitely.

2. An anti-inflammatory low or zero carb meat-based diet will optimize ozone treatments. At the very least, sugars, gluten, and most grains should be eliminated.

3. It is a good idea to have a backup plan when performing DIV ozone injections since if they are performed long term they will sooner or later result in damaged veins. Veins can sclerose, collapse, or develop scar tissue. This can make it impossible or very difficult to inject them in the future. Even the most pronounced veins can collapse if they are punctured too many times and at high enough ozone concentrations. Which is why it is advisable to keep other ozone options open like ozone saunas, drinking ozonated water, or do ozone insufflations.

4. The rationale why ozone therapy could theoretically have anti-cancer properties is that just like chemotherapy or radiation it could lead to a fatal increase of ROS (reactive oxygen species) inside tumor cells.

Chapter 18 answers

1. A Herxheimer reaction is also called a healing crisis, a die-off, or a detox reaction.

    It describes the resurgence of symptoms while pathogens are killed off. It is assumed that this happens because of endotoxins which are released when certain bacteria die.

2. There is no bullet-proof way to distinguish an ozone induced Herxheimer reaction from an adverse reaction. But there are a few indications which can point towards it:

    - a first improvement directly after the ozone treatment followed by a worsening. That worsening can be the herx.
    - If the worsening after the last ozone treatment can be lessened or resolved with subsequent ozone treatments, then this points towards a herx.

    - If after the resolution of the symptoms which have emerged directly after the ozone treatments, a new level of well-being emerges which was not there before the ozone treatments.

    - If there is an emergence of old symptoms after ozone treatments which were believed to be long gone and if those symptoms get triggered after each new ozone treatment.

- The emergence of fever, feeling like coming down with the flu, nasal discharge, coughing up phlegm, increased need for sleep, rashes, achiness in joints

3. The following is a list of ideas how to deal with ozone induced herxheimer reactions:

- Drink ozonated water
- Do more ozone treatments. It sounds counterintuitive, but often more ozone treatments can resolve the Herxheimer reaction which was triggered by ozone treatments.
- Take several grams of vitamin C
- Do less ozone treatments: either reduce the frequency, or reduce the ozone concentration, or the duration of the ozone treatments.
- Wait it out, allow time to pass.

Chapter 19 answers

1. As of the writing of this book, Dr. Robins claims to have performed around 310,000 DIVs in his practice in New York City without a single known fatality.

2. In the past 60 years several million oxyvenierung treatments have been performed in Germany, also without a single known fatality.

3. There are 19 well-documented cases of people having died after drinking too much water, around 14 more than are attributed to DIV ozone injections.

4. It is estimated that between 150 and 500 people die each year in the US due to Tylenol, and around 7,600 due to NSAIDs like aspirin.

Made in the USA
Las Vegas, NV
16 March 2024